Pills, Thrills and Methadone Spills 2: Techs, Drugs and Birth Control

By Mr Dispenser

Contents

4

Foreword

To say it is an absolute honour and delight to be asked to provide a short foreword to Mr Dispenser's second and yet again highly entertaining book is quite an understatement. For someone who is still trying to come to terms with Facebook, tweeting or using social media was never ever going to be for me. However it was only after meeting Mr Dispenser, that I was introduced to the phenomenal world of Twitter. Today I would NEVER be without it thanks to Mr Dispenser.

This current edition of Pills, Thrills and Methadone Spills 2 fails to disappoint once again, engaging its audience in masses with ever-growing popularity. It continues to capture the reality of pharmacy and its practice through a satirical but almost addictive mist of tweets, which constantly surface through the twittersphere with better predictive regularity than a good dose of senna. Having endless reach using only 140 characters, the book cleverly demonstrates just how much fun pharmacy is and importantly the immeasurable power of social media.

Mr Dispenser has now tip toed into America with his books and no doubt is aspiring to capture America almost like the Beatles in the '60s? His superb collection of witty reality in the daily lives of pharmacists from all sectors can be compelling to many. Interestingly, his knowledge of pharmacy from both professional and legal quarters allows him to humour and even inform many of his 1000s of followers in more ways than one.

Before the day has even begun and the pharmacy shutters are pulled up ready for business, Mr Dispenser awakens many of his followers with his first morning anecdotes. To some locum pharmacists trying to have a lie-in, this may appear like having breakfast in bed with the daily rag! He pools in the knowledge of some very clever and highly experienced healthcare professionals. At the end of a hard day's work in the pharmacy and the shutters are pulled down he soon takes off to his twittersphere. Mr Dispenser then emerges in full strength often pitting his wits against the cream of the crop but always ensuring he disappears again with the last tweet before bedtime for many to ponder on.

In this book, Mr Dispenser's addiction is also revealed through his craving for pens – typically exposing the real life community pharmacist blood in him! Furthermore he has grown in confidence so much that now you can read about Mr Dispenser's own law. He has even started 'tweeting tips' for new doctors, not to mention his skirting with motivational and inspirational theories – almost as if he was a behavioural social guru. The funniest is when he believes he is the twitter master of chat-up lines. Meanwhile his Christmas Pharmacy lyrics somehow give me the feeling he may be challenging for the next Christmas number one – look out Bing Crosby!

A fascinating vision of everyday pharmacy with a light hearted awakening – a truly wonderful compilation that readers from all walks of life, and from within the pharmacy profession from students, to practitioners to academics, will all find a must read book. Social media has allowed him to reach out further than one's imagination as it did for me, probably the world's biggest anti-social media person at one point.

Finally it's great to support the fact that some of the proceeds will be going to charity as with the first book and I wholeheartedly wish Mr Dispenser every success for the future.

Dr Mahendra G Patel, RPS Board Member

Preface

So here we are again. The first book was published in January 2013 and it was more popular than I had ever envisaged. I was overwhelmed by the response, which, along with generous contributions from friends and followers who are too numerous to mention, spurred me on. A second book appeared to be a formality.

This second volume contains more contributions gathered via social media, for which I make no apologies. Social media did after all help me to create the first book and played a large part in making it a success. It was Franklin Roosevelt who said that, 'The only thing we have to fear is...fear itself': I'm pretty sure he was talking about social media.

Although @MrDodgyChemist once said to a patient, 'If I could ask you to not stand there please. It's a breach of confidentiality. You could easily see my Facebook password from there.' I would encourage all pharmacy personnel to use social media to talk to each other.

Again, I would like to thank Lucy Pitt and The Pharmacy Show team for their wonderful support. My thanks also go to Richard Daniszewski, Laura Shaw and Kirsty Hough for their proof-reading.

I do sometimes forget about all the contributions and call them 'my' books. This is wrong: They are 'OUR' books. Please enjoy responsibly and don't read it whilst patients are waiting for their prescription. Unless, of course, they complain about the waiting time, in which case read it out loud.

There are no plans currently for a third book and I don't have enough material anyway. If this is the end, then I am happy with the way it ended.

Again 5% of sales are going to the Pharmacist Support Charity.

Signing out as Responsible Pharmacist

Mr Dispenser

@MrDodgyChemist: You know you use Twitter too much when a patient asks you a question about their medicines and you check twitter for interactions and not the BNF.

Being Early

What reasons have you had had for a patient requesting their medicines earlier than expected? E.g. my dog ate my tablets.

1] Steve T: Not really on-topic, but I once took a call from a lady who told me that her husband had passed away. After offering her our condolences she asked if she could continue to order his pills as she *"likes taking some of them"*...

2] Andy C: *"It was raining when I picked up my prescription and they got wet so I put them in the microwave to dry out. Apparently you're not supposed to put foil in the microwave."*

3] Carley E: *"I ran over my DDS pack in my electric wheel chair."*

4] David R: We must have dispensed them short last time it's the only explanation! (All 26 items).

5] Katie S: Going on holiday for 2 weeks then see them in town the following week.

6] Sarah W: *"The pack was empty - you dispensed an empty pack."*

7] Anna D: A few years ago now but I had a wife come in asking for more of her husband's Zimovane LS tablets as she had thought they were Viagra and flushed them down the toilet. She realised her mistake the following night when her husband said he couldn't find his sleeping tablets so did she fancy a bit of fun instead...

8] Sandra G: *"It's my birthday!"* (Viagra).

9] Conchetta L: *"I was on a boat, but unfortunately the boat sank, along with my Vicodin."*

10] Claire S: *"You didn't hand my medicines to me when I signed for them."*

11] Debbie F: *"I put them in the recycling bin."*

12] Tina S: *"I got burgled."*

13] Adam P: *"I threw the zopiclone in the fire because I thought it was just the cardboard box and I burn all my cardboard boxes."*

14] Barbara P: *"I left the bag on the bus."*

15] Susan F: *"A seagull swooped down and took my fentanyl patches!"*

16] Amanda H: *"Someone must have stolen them from my trolley."*

17] Naomi S: *"Dog ate my tablets out of a MDS tray."*

18] @Dj_rai: *"I'm going to court in the morning."*

19] @AmandaHepburn88*: "I kept my effervescent co-codamol under the sink and they got wet."*

20] @SamRaybould: *"I left them on a helicopter!"*

21] @BCLPF: *"I went into hospital and the ward lost my inhaler."*

22] @surveyor53: *"The police stopped me last night, took all my pills, here's the bottles I need refilled."*

23] @rxshane*:"My ferret took my prescription bottle and hid them from me."* Two things I didn't believe: the excuse...and the gall to claim such crap!

24] @rxshane: *"My cat knocked my bottle of Norcos into the sink and down the drain."*

25] @Lolaskates: *"My grandson flushed my furosemide down the toilet!"*

26] @Pharm_Thoughts: *"I let my son play with my MDI inhaler because his squirt gun was broken."*

27] Andy C: Excuses I've heard regarding asking for benzodiazepines early include:

"You gave me an empty box."

"The foil strip was empty."

"You never put them in my bag."

"They were the wrong shape so I threw them in the bin."

"The canary ate them."

"The tablets broke every time I popped them out the foil."

"They were stolen out my pocket."

"They've been put on the top shelf in the kitchen and I can't reach them."

"I accidentally flushed them away when I went to the toilet."

"My grandson fed them to the ducks."

Doses

1] @dansmith109: *"FOUR 5ml spoonful's into the vagina!"* Messy and ineffective way of using Epilim!

2] @OakfieldNo6: When typing PRN accidentally hitting an O and printing out PORN.

3] @Sexy_in-scrubs: A script for a male patient once said to insert ONE tablet per vagina. And it was for something like Crestor!

4] @himalmakwana: *"Instil ONE drop into the rectum FOUR times daily."* Chloramphenicol Eye Drops.

5] @Mrsfinn86: *"Insert ONE in each vagina".* I see this error every week printed out on prescriptions. It still makes me laugh.

6] @Susie_Harvey: *"Take ONE TREE times a day".*

7] @pokey_pineapple: Viagra. *"Take ONE tablet by mouth when horny."* But that was on purpose.

8] @Vento: *"ONE to be taken one hour before anticipated romance".*

9] @ArvindSami91: On a label for suppositories. *"Take ONE in the arse."*

10] @a_lethal_dose: Our system will generate a HAPPY NEW YEAR direction. No lie.

11] @SparklyStacey88: On a prescription from a GP for a cream *"As directed by spermatologist".*

12] Louise M: Canesten...*"Apply to Volvo THREE times a day".*

13] Ailidh N: *"Use as a soup substitute!"*

14] Graham S: *"Apply to family jewels."*

15] Sally S: *"Take when hungry"* on Juvela loaves!

16] Lesley R: Yesterday Co-codamol 8/500mg *"Take 102 tablets FOUR times a day".*

17] Rosemarie A: For Nitrolingual *"Use ONE spray to the right eye!"*

18] Wendy F: I once received diazepam 5mg labelled as *"Take as directed - do not eat them all at once or you will miss your holiday."*

19] Adam C: *"TWO puffs when required via Facebook".* (Apparently she meant via face mask).

20] Martin M: For diclofenac suppositories- *"Insert THREE times a day with food."*

21] Maria R: *"ONE TWICE a day till death."*

22] Reena G: *"Insert FIVE prednisolone suppositories each morning for exacerbation of asthma."*

23] Stephen S: *"Take 5ml prior to haircut!?"*

24] James T: For Ventolin inhaler *"Spray one puff inserted high into the vagina when required."*

25] Vicky C: Optrex Infected eye drops- *"Instil one drop FOUR times daily under foreskin."*

26] Joanna H: *"Inhale half a puff."*

27] Paul F: On amoxicillin, *"Take ONE three times daily for five days then return unused medicine to the pharmacy."* Supply 21 capsules. From out of hours surgery.

28] @lil_ms_cheesey: I had a repeat prescription come through with the *directions "lazy doctor never checks before signing!"* (it was signed!).

29] @Missimmy: Atenolol 25mg-*"Take NONE in the morning".* I think they meant ONE.

30] @lil_ms_cheesey: Best one I've had was clopidogrel, supply ONE tab. *"5mls THREE times a day".* Receptionist couldn't understand the problem!

31] Lisa C: 28 furosemide 40mg - fine you say? Dosage - Take one every second!

Chat Up Lines

1] @MrDispenser: Is it me or is there an interaction between us?

2] @MrDodgyChemist: 'Is this a new medication?' 'No.' 'Ok, in that case can I have your phone number anyway?'

3] @ZainyBebe: "Lucky for you I'm Thick 'n' Easy"!!

4] Lisa J K: Apply me to your sensitive area.

5] Stephen S: Would you prefer something to suck on?

6] @bbbbarrel: I think I can stop my risedronate from now on because you have significantly increased my bone strength

7] Shikha R-T: Is your name flecainide? Cause u just made my heart skip a beat.

8] Martin P: Put your white coat on, you've pulled.

9] @ArvindSami91: You need to add me to methadone register, because I'm addicted to you

10] @MrDispenser: I have sugar free methadone because I'm sweet enough.

11] @LoopyShaw: Do you fraudulently sign the back of your scripts as you got FINE written all over you?

12] @MrDodgyChemist: 'Wow! That was so quick!' said the lady as I gave out her prescription. 'How about I show you something even quicker tonight?'

13] @MrDodgyChemist: 'It's just one tablet and best taken with food, ASAP. So how about I buy you dinner and you can take it then?'

14] @MrDodgyChemist: I'm old, single and ready for shingles

15] @MrDodgyChemist: 'Would you and your partner be interested in a free Chlamydia test? Oh, you are single? Yeah I will go out with you then.'

Dubious Pharmacy Facts

1] @MrDispenser: Methadone is also available as a brand called *'I can't believe it's not Methadone'.* This has fewer calories.

2] @kevfrost: Pharmacies in the jungle constantly run out of aspirin. The parrots eat 'em all. (C) The League of Gentlemen.

3] @MrDispenser: The GP's wife is never the practice manager.

4] @MrDispenser: Pharmacies love to get phone calls asking if they are open.

5] @The_Buffy_Bot: When we don't have your medicine in stock we nip down to Boots and get it from them.

6] @MrDispenser: Amoxicillin tablets exist and the correct dose is FOUR times daily.

7] @rmoomin1: The fizzy co-codamol in the foil packets are the only ones that work. Fizzy co-codamol in paper packets are imposters.

8] @MrDispenser: I never tweet at work.

9] @drgandalf52: There is a secret room where they keep the 'good' drugs. Oh wait, that's true!

10] @MrDispenser: Orlistat was never out of stock. We just think that fat people are more jolly.

11] @The_Buffy_Bot: Any uncollected drugs go into a hamper that's then raffled off at the Christmas party.

12] @drgandalf52: There is an elf that steals all the pens attached to wires at a pharmacy desk. He is called P. Atients.

13] @aye_sure: Pharmacist's don't wait until their CPD is called to write it all up!

14] @drgandalf52: When they run out of inhalers, they refill the old ones with Glade Plug and Fresh. This cures asthma and bad breath.

15] @The_Buffy_Bot: When you become a pharmacist you never have to pay a prescription charge ever again.

16] @MrDispenser: Doctors never forget to sign a prescription and always check what's on it before signing.

17] @The_Buffy_Bot: GP receptionists are medically trained professionals.

18] @weeneldo: Illegal supply of a class A drug? Could do life for it. But I'm not an expert; I'm a pharmacist, not a receptionist.

19] @The_Buffy_Bot: We know exactly which medicines you are taking from the description "It's a little round white pill".

20] @NavinSewak: OTC medicines are effective.

21] @cocksparra: The nurse prescribers have magical scripts. They can prescribe you dressings in ANY size you like, ANY size.

22] @NavinSewak: Pharmacies have everything in stock, all the time. It's their job to do so.

23] @NavinSewak: Doctors understand the role of the pharmacist.

24] @TheCynicalRPh: Pharmacists understand the role of the pharmacist.

25] @The_Buffy_Bot: Pharmacists aren't really necessary because doctors get prescriptions right every time.

Top Pharmacy Lies

1] @thingsaboutemmy: *"Of course I know it's only for short term use."*

2] @BumperPMP: *"We will, of course, provide you with every possible support from Head Office to help you to achieve your annual MUR target."*

3] @LouiseAliceX: *"Oh yeah, of course I'm taking co-codamol for 3 days only."*

4] @Mexican_Badger: *"No, I have never purchased Solpadeine Max before."*

5] @josh6h: *"My doctor says.."*

6] @googlybear84: *"Yes these tablets are for someone else."*

7] @shalpatz: *"I dropped my prescription somewhere but I can tell you what's on it."*

8] @shalpatz: *"I'm not buying this medication for my dog."*

9] @shalpatz: *"I won't use the hydrocortisone cream on my face."*

10] @sue_warman: When giving out metronidazole – *"I don't drink."*

11] @sue_warman: *"I have been at home all day* (but the delivery driver carded you!).

12] @sue_warman: *"I have emptied everything out of the bag and it's definitely not in there."*

13] @Cleverestcookie: *"No I didn't change the quantity from 28 to 280."*

14] @EmilyJaneBond82: *"I've always bought metoclopramide over the counter from here."*

15] @pill_saurus: *"We will give you a ring once your item is in stock!"*

16] @EmilyJaneBond82: *"I ordered my prescription and was told it would be ready this morning."*

17] @Cleverestcookie: *"No, I don't take any other tablets... (Except those rat poison ones, but they don't count)."*

18] @pill_saurus: *"The other pharmacy always gives me that brand!"*

19] @theancientartof: *"I'm a doctor in my own country and I definitely need some cyclizine."*

20] @Cleverestcookie: *"Yes, I always follow the pharmacist's advice, even though they just count Smarties."*

21] @MykelO: *"I always get my prescriptions here."* (PMR shows mainly emergency supplies).

22] @theancientartof: *"The paramedic I called out last night for an asthma attack. They definitely said it was ok NOT to use my brown inhaler. Can I have a Ventolin?"*

23] @pill_saurus: *"Can I have some co-codamol? I use it occasionally for back pain."*

24] @theancientartof: *"My GP definitely said I could buy diazepam without a prescription."*

25] @MrDispenser: *"I'll bring my warfarin book in next time."*

26] @Zahel: *"The wholesaler let us down"* (we didn't forget to order it in time honest).

27] @Zahel: *"I can't wait 20 minutes for my prescription I have a bus to catch!"*

28] @himalmakwana: *"I carry my Ventolin with me at all times."*

29] @MrDispenser: Customer: *"Can I buy some Medised please?"*

Me*: "How old is the child?"*

Customer: *"Six."*

30] @jobiwhan: *"I've completed a stock count and it is 100% correct."*

31] @alkemist1912: *"I only take Nytol occasionally."*

32] @alkemist1912: *"I want some Phenergan for travel sickness for my 8 year old."*

33] @alkemist1912: *"I'm not on any other medication."*

Pharmacy Games

1] Deborah L: I once wheeled myself from the clinical checking bench (in the olden days of course) to the CD room using only an armrest support (unfortunately passed an outpatient at the hatch at the time!); got caught having a sword fight with said armrests by the dispensary manager (she was NOT happy!); and used to (note the "used to") play practical jokes on them all.

2] Katie H: Find the script!

3] Si B: Dare a staff member to sneak in a random word or noise whilst talking to a customer, and hope that they don't pick up on it.

4] Ann P: The psychiatric hospital with the BNF order dispensary taught me a great game: Promazine cricket. Pre-pack bottle of 50 Promazine tablets bowled across dispensary and smacked as hard as possible with a plank of wood. The winner was the person who eventually made the bottle explode and the (bright blue) tablets go everywhere. Hours of fun. That was also the hospital where I learned to make paracetamol bombs: if you've worked for me, I've probably taught you to do this. If not, forget I mentioned it and move on: nothing to see here...

5] @SparkleWildfire: The "How many Calcichew D3 Forte can you fit in a bottle?" game.

6] @drgandalf: See a better game is how many Calcichew D3 Forte can you fit in your mouth?

7] Rani R: You have time to play games?

8] Samia N: We play "guess what that patient heading straight towards us is going to ask?"

9] Jo B: Decipher the handwritten prescription.

10] Anwen B: Spot the Levonelle customer as they walk through the door! Brilliant in a student area!

11] Priya J: "Chair game"- back in the day when it was quiet!! Sit on wheeled chair and see how far across dispensary you could push yourself (not compliant with Health and Safety me thinks!)

12] Angela C: Guess where the bag of dispensed medicines has been filed?!

13] Becky W: I play the yes/no game with what drug am I? Everyone hates it but me! But it teaches them about medication!

14] Jo B: Water fights with oral syringes.

15] Richard H: Best game I play is 'can I drink some of this coffee before I get called to the counter and it goes stone cold?'. I think I managed it once. It was a Wednesday.

16] Gina E: One of the dispensers hid in a large box and saw who she could jump out and surprise (long waits when customers were in and we had to work), only the wholesaler delivery guy fell for it. Nearly gave him a heart attack. Those were the days...

17] Yasmina H: Rock, paper, scissors on who has to answer the phone next!

18] Ricky H: I like to play "give the locum a hard time."

19] Lisa F: How long you can hold a Martindale..

20] Carley E: A fellow dispenser and I used to shout out a drug name, then the other had to say another drug that starts with the last letter of the first drug. Not only fun trying to think of one but also the look on everyone else's face that has no idea what we are doing or what condition the patient has that we are discussing!! Citalopram, Mebendazole., Elleste Solo, Oramorph, etc.

21] Hayley B: We play guess the delivery drivers name. It's 20p a go. Whoever gets it wins the money or doesn't pay into the tea kitty for that week... We seem to have a new AAH driver every week.

MY BLOGS 1

Pens for Pharmacy Charity

Dear Pharmacy colleague,

Now in existence for over 1/7 days, Pens for Pharmacy continues to strive to expand its programs and offerings to the community. We hope that you will be able to take part in one or more of the many exciting events that we are offering this year and experience first-hand the pride we take in supporting our cause.

It is our mission to ensure that every pharmacy has enough pens. We have had reports of some pharmacies sharing one pen. Clearly, this is unacceptable. In order to meet our mission and provide services in our community, we rely on the generosity of individuals and businesses for support. Without the assistance of community-minded individuals just like you, we wouldn't be able to help those in our pharmacies each year.

We ask that you make a commitment to support our annual appeal by making a pen donation. This year our goal is 5 pens for each pharmacy, and we hope that you will be able to make a contribution. Your generosity will make a difference in our community by allowing us to continue in our work. If you give one pen to a pharmacy, then research shows that they will lose it within 20 minutes. If you give them 5 pens, then it will be 5 times longer before they lose it.

We have enclosed a donor envelope for your convenience. Remember that every pen makes a difference, regardless of colour, size or drug name. The look on the faces of the little technicians when you give them a pen is heart-warming.

Thank you in advance for your support!

Sincerely,

Mr Dispenser, CEO, Pens for Pharmacy Charity

Mr Dispenser's Law

Have you heard of Mr Dispenser's Law? I'm sure you have. It states that if something can go wrong it will go wrong. Unfortunately it always happens to the same patient, poor Mr Smith!

Here are ten reasons why we were unable to deliver his medicines.

1] His Oilatum was unavailable last year for months. He didn't believe me.

2] His isosorbide mononitrate was unavailable due to an explosion at the factory. He didn't believe me.

3] The fridge failed so we were unable to supply his Proctosedyl suppositories. He didn't believe me.

4] His Wockhardt generic medicines got recalled by the manufacturer. He didn't believe me.

5] The wholesaler sent the wrong item. He didn't believe me.

6] The wholesaler driver got a flat tyre so was unable to come that day. He didn't believe me.

7] His Cialis was on quota. He didn't believe me.

8] His prescription was waiting to be signed by the doctor. He didn't believe me.

9] After six years of him waiting in the shop with his 20 item script, we persuaded him to sign up to the reorder scheme and get his medication delivered. It snowed. Our driver couldn't deliver. He didn't believe me.

10] We were shut on Christmas Day and Boxing Day. He didn't believe me.

The Show Must Go On!

There are ten things that are designed to stop the workflow in a pharmacy:

1] Babies: I love babies. I used to be one. But they hate work. They must do.

2] Former staff coming to visit: Catching up with those who have left slows us down. We never spoke to them while they were here. That's why they left.

3] Former staff coming to visit who have had babies: See points one and two and then double them.

4] Twitter: It stops me working. I'll explain more once I check the prescription that's waiting.

5] Patients: Yes, I know we need them but things would happen quicker if they did not interrupt us and ask when the next bus into town is coming.

6] The weekend: Monday morning should be renamed 'Spending the whole morning talking about what happened on the weekend'. No work gets done.

7] Area managers: Everybody works slower as they walk on egg shells and hope they don't get asked a question about targets.

8] Love life: Once we have explored the reasons why the counter assistant got dumped by the milkman, then work can commence.

9] Tea: This is a vital part of the workplace but when you have 6 cups a day and 6 staff then it takes one poor individual 30 minutes of the day to make it.

10] Reality TV: OMG, why did Gary Barlow vote off the lady who made that cake from Strictly? I think I have got that right.

Handing out a prescription

Checking is easy; handing out a prescription is the hard part. Some people don't even let me ask for their address before they tell me it. This saddens me. I like my routine. It's highly embarrassing when I randomly change the patient's sex due to oversight on the name. Who knew that handing out a prescription could be so emotional?

I handed out a prescription. The patient said, *"That was quick"*. I said, *"That's what Mrs Dispenser says..."*

Sometimes I shout out patient's names and they just say 'Yes' and sit there. Unless, you're really old, heavily pregnant, good looking, in a wheelchair or have given me a pen in the past, I don't come to you. One guy actually put his hand up when I shouted his name. This is now in the SOP.

I handed out a prescription to Mr Smith. I said, *"This medication needs to be taken with food."* Mrs Smith who was also there said: *"Don't worry. He doesn't need any encouragement to eat..."*

"Prescription for Mrs Smith" Mr Smith: *"21 Coronation St. Well, she was there when I left the house!"* I said: *"Hopefully, she'll still be there when you get back"* Mr Smith: *"Easy for you to say. You don't live with her!"*

41

Ever had twins? Two people with the same name waiting at same time and both come up to collect script! It was surreal.

Every so often I ask for the date of birth instead of address when handing out prescriptions. It confuses the hell out of people.

I shout out the name. No one answers. I shout again. No one answers. A patient shouts his name in case I am thick and can't read. I shout name again. Then another patient decides to help and starts shouting it out and asking everyone else if it's them.

I hate it when you ask for their address and they go to grab the bag without telling you. You don't let go until they tell you. Prescription tug of war!

I asked a patient to confirm his address. He turned around and pointed at the house across the street. The house number and the street name were clearly visible.

I asked a lady to confirm her address and she said that she's not telling me. I gave her my patented "I haven't got time for this shit" look.

If I wasn't a pharmacist, I'd be doing Shakespeare on stage. I've learnt to project when shouting out people's names. It is awkward though when you shout out a patient's name and they are standing next to you and startle you.

Sometimes, no one has told me that the patient is calling back and I shout louder and louder. I then have to put the prescription in the right alphabet box. No one gave us any training on this at university. They foolishly believed that we knew our alphabet. My inability to put checked prescriptions in appropriate alphabet box is legendary. It's hard!

What They Say and What They Mean

1] WTS: Your prescription is ready. It just needs checking by the pharmacist

WTM: The pharmacist is slow as hell

2] WTS: Dispensing is a complicated process and takes time. It's not as easy as slapping a label on a box

WTM: The dispensers need to discuss last night's Coronation Street first

3] WTS: Could you please change this Oxycontin 5mg MR to the Oxybutynin 5mg MR prescribed please?

WTM: I'm not working here again

4] WTS: I was late to work due to traffic

WTM: I woke up late

5] WTS: Hi, welcome to the pharmacy, we love locums

WTM: You better do some MURs or we will spit in your tea

6] WTS: I know we said that your medication would be ready today but the wholesalers messed up

WTM: We forgot to order it

7] WTS: I just need to clarify something with the doctor

WTM: I can't read the doctor's handwriting

8] WTS: Sorry for the delay with your prescription, we are having computer issues

WTM: Susan has managed to misplace your prescription

9] WTS: Your prescription is ready but we just need to locate it

WTM: The pharmacist has alphabet issues and has put it in the wrong box

10] WTS: Your prescription is with the driver and is on it's way

WTM: Oh crap, ring Alan and tell him to come back and pick up this delivery

11] WTS: My CPD record is up to date

WTM: I will start when I'm called up

12] WTS: I only have one biscuit with my tea

WTM: I have four biscuits with my tea

13] WTS: I haven't stolen your pen

WTM: I have stolen your pen

14] WTS: You rang to ask if we're open. No, that's not a stupid question.

WTM: That's a stupid question

Mexican Stand-Off

"I've come to collect my prescription"

"Ok…"

So it begins. The Mexican Stand-Off. I refuse to ask her what her name is and she refuses to tell me. The staring starts. Never breaking eye contact. Not once. Ok, maybe once when I respond to the 'Who wants a cuppa?' question.

I have all the time in the world. Actually, I don't. But she doesn't know that. She thinks she knows me. She thinks she's the expert on me. She isn't.

I know her name. Of course. I see her all the time. She knows that I know her name. But I shouldn't have to ask her what her name is. If I do, she has won.

I can't allow that to happen. I must make a stand for everyone who has ever worked in a pharmacy and been faced with the same situation. I must not surrender. Not now, not ever.

Susan the Tech: *"For crying out loud Mr D. Must we go through this every time she comes in? Just give your mum her prescription and let's get back to work, eh?"*

Damn you Susan! I was sure I would win this time!

Staff Night Out

After our first Staff Night Out, we decided to try again but order a takeaway this time and go back to my house and watch a DVD. I was looking forward to relaxing after another day with difficult patients.

I had not ordered before I got to the takeaway. I went in and said that it was quiet. There was a chorus of groans from the staff because I said the Q word! I asked if it would be long because I had a taxi waiting.

I leant on the counter and did not step away the whole time. I was asked to have a seat but I ignored them. One of the dispensers wanted to go large on her burger meal but wanted diet coke as she had a Weight Watchers meeting the next day.

A guy came in and was very mad. He said that he had just received a delivery and that they had tried to poison him! They had given him chilli sauce instead of tomato sauce. This had happened before and he was going to report them. The assistant looked at the receipt and replied that it was not her that had done it.

As I got my food, I checked it in front of the assistant before I left, to make sure it was right. Luckily for them it was. On my way out, I saw one of the staff clearing the tables and noticed that half the food had been left on one of the tables. What a waste! I was glad that I did not work there.

POP CULTURE 1

Pharmacy TV

1] **@MrDispenser**: Downton Abilify

2] **@i_Q_Balls:** Pharmacy Break- A Pharmacist's brother attempts to break him out of a long 100 hour shift

3] **@Calorinee:** Big Bang Theophylline

4] **@MrDispenser**: Law and Dispensary Order

5] **@rikash_p:** Great British Bandage Off

6] **@MrDispenser**: Saved by the Belladonna Plaster

7] **@Calorinee:** Hibiscrubs

8] **@MrDispenser**: ALFuzosin

9] **@FlitmanJ**: Top Gear

10] **@MrDispenser:** Magnum Parallel Import

11] **@aptaim:** R*A*S*H

12] **@aptaim:** The Fresh Prince of Fostair

13] **@Cleverestcookie:** The One-Alpha Show

14] **@MrDispenser:** Nytol Rider

15] **@mawellings:** Never mind the Fluclox

16] @MrDispenser: Diff'rent types of Strokes

17] @MrDispenser: I'm a Locum, get me out of here

18] @OneMissSharan: Strictly Come Dispensing

19] @pharma_ali: In the Nytol garden

20] @MrDispenser: Doctor Who? I can't make out the signature!

21] @henrysjl: The Rx Factor

22] @georgiasalter: Questran Time

23] @MrsLynneJ: Sex and the Citalopram

24] @cathrynjbrown: How I Methadone Your Mother

25] @CrackedPestle: Solostar Trek

26] @MrDispenser: Fe Side

27] @CrackedPestle: "60 Minims"

28] @pharma_ali: Have I got Muse for you

29] @pharma_ali: The Big Bong Theory

30] @weeneldo: The Only Way is Ethics

31] @Pharm_Thoughts: Once Upon a 15 minute wait Time

32] @Pharm_Thoughts: Teen Moms 4: the Plan B edition

33] **@Sengad:** Guys and Tramadols

34] **@pharma_ali:** Sex and the Cialis

35] **@rikash_p:** The Big Boots Theory

36] **@georgiasalter:** The Weakest Linctus

37] **@georgiasalter:** Geordie Ensure

38] **@kelbel69696969:** Constipation Street

39] **@tnyone2:** Dancing on NICE

40] **@dthaker06:** The Xalatan factor

Films about Pharmacy

1] The Running Man: Chasing people who have not paid for their prescriptions

2] The Hunger Games: Time for elevenses

3] This Means War: Another pharmacy opens down the road

4] Mean Girls: Staff ganging up on one member of staff

5] Taken: My pen gets stolen

6] Usual Suspects: The same people always steal my pen

7] Horrible Bosses: No one likes their manager

8] Training Day: Work Experience

9] The Good, The Bad and The Ugly: Pharmacy staff

10] Some Like it Hot: Tea and Coffee

11] There Will Be Blood: Flu vaccination

12] The Great Escape: Sneaking off to the toilet

Star Wars Guide to Pharmacy

Pharmacy has a lot in common with Star Wars.

1] @JonnyB_at_RMP: Ever met a Jedi GP receptionist? *"These are not the scripts you are looking for."*

2] @MrDispenser: GP Yoda says, *"The correct dose it is"*.

3] @LSD_Locums: Darth Patient says, *"I want you to search it again; I am not leaving without my prescription"*.

4] @JonnyB_at_RMP: The AAH delivery van is running late again: the fastest hunk o' junk in the galaxy!

5] @LSD_Locums: GPhC Emperor says. *'"You scruffy pharmacists are no match for the power of my epic lawsuit and threat of closure."*

6] @MrDispenser: Jabba the Hut is upset that Orlistat is out of stock.

7] @LSD_Locums: Bowsk the bounty hunter is annoyed because there are still problems with Oilatum..

8] @MrDispenser: Qui-Gon Jinn the pre-reg tutor is keeping an eye on Anakin the Pre-reg.

9] @MrDispenser: R2-D2 the pharmacy robot has broken down again.

10] @LSD_Locums: C-3PO the area manager has come to chat about missing targets.

11] @MrDispenser: Han Solo the locum is late again.

12] @LSD_Locums: And he texts his mate Lando about working in his shop one day.

13] @JonnyB_at_RMP: How about the Republic's latest treatment for osteoporosis, R-chew D-3?

14] @LSD_Locums: Would there be an NRT called Chewbacca?

15] @JonnyB_at_RMP: Personally, I'm still looking for the 'Small thermal exhaust port' on the side of Boots head office.

16] @PharmakeusPrime: "You practiced in that dispensary? You're braver than I thought!"

17] @LSD_Locums: "I am NOT a formulary!"

18] @PharmakeusPrime: "The MPharm Course is what gives a pharmacist their powers. It's like an energy field that unites us".

19] @LSD_Locums: We forgot Superintendent Leia.

20] @PharmakeusPrime: You have learned much prereg. But you are not a pharmacist yet.

21] @LSD_Locums: *"If you fire me now, I will become more powerful than you could possibly imagine".*

22] @PharmakeusPrime: Luke, I know we booked you for the Hoth branch but we need you to work in the Dagobah branch instead.

23] @LSD_Locums: Pharmacy owner Tarkin to Superintendent Leia: *"You don't know how hard I found it, signing over your shares".*

24] @PharmakeusPrime: I'm amazed you had the courage to sign off these SOPs yourself.

25] @PharmakeusPrime: So you have a twin sister. If you won't work for Lloyd's, maybe she will?

26] @PharmakeusPrime: Evacuation ? At our moment of triumph? Could the Picolax not have waited?

27] @dressage_diva: Luke, use the force of the spray twice a day.

28] @PharmakeusPrime: I used to bullseye 25ml bottles into a T6 carton back home.

29] @JohnnyB_at_RMP: I heard medicines optimisation was just a 'hokey religion'.

30] @MrDispenser: A long time ago in a dispensary far far away, it turned out that the guy with heavy breathing had COPD.

31] @aamersafdar: Pre-reg who qualifies and locums in your pharmacy: *'When I left you, I was the learner, now I'm the master.'*

32] @aamersafdar: Pharmacist to store manager obsessed with MUR targets: *'Do not succumb to the dark side.'*

33] @aamersafdar: Good new pre-reg arrives: *'The force is strong with this one.'*

Pharmacy Films

1] **@sarayummymummy:** Puss in Boots.

2] **@kevfrost:** MHRA Class 1: Total Recall.

3] **@Cleverestcookie:** Four Errors and a Funeral.

4] **@googlybear84:** Sleepless in Cialis.

5] **@vento:** Lyclear and Present Danger.

6] **@veto:** EPS I love you.

7] **@vento:** To Kill Amoxil Bird.

8] **@vento:** A Hard Day's Nitrate.

9] **@ShabnamMirza:** Scary Movicol.

10] **@vento:** Dianette Another Day.

11] **@s9njay:** Risedronate of the Planet of the Apes.

12] **@vento:** NMS of the State.

13] **@alkemist1912:** Galaxy Questran.

14] **@vento:** Who Framed Roger Rabipur?

15] **@alkemist:** The Spy who came in with a cold.

16] **@iPothecary:** Dr No (I won't let you join the CCG).

17] **@vento:** Ali Baba and The Fortisip Thieves.

18] @MrDispenser: Lorenzo's Oilatum.

19] @vento: I Know What You Did Last Sumatriptan.

20] @pgimmo: Live and Let Direct Supply.

21] @vento: The Maxtrex.

22] @kevfrost: On Her Majesty's Prescription Delivery Service.

23] @pgimmo: Never Say Teva Again.

24] @kevfrost: The Man with The Cold Sores Gum.

25] @pill_O_Saurus_: Durogesic Park.

9-5

Tumble out of bed and stumble to the kitchen;

Pour myself a cup of ambition,

And yawn, and stretch, and try to come to life.

Jump in the shower, and the blood starts pumping;

Out on the street, the traffic Starts jumping,

With folks like me on the job from nine to five.

Working nine to five thirty, staying behind to enter CDs, what a way to make a living;

Department of health, it's all taking and no giving.

AAH sends you the wrong stuff and they never give you credit;

It's enough to drive you crazy, if you let it.

Nine to six, for enhanced service and devotion;

also throwing in some health promotion;

want some more staff, but the area manager won't seem to let me.

I swear sometimes, that man is out to get me.

They give you unrealistic targets, just to see hope your hopes shatter;

You're just a step on the Boots ladder,

But you've got dreams he'll never take away.

In the same boat with a lot of your colleagues;

Waitin' on the day your orlistat will come In,

And the tide's gonna turn, and you'll do two MURs a day.

Working nine to six thirty, staying behind to do paperwork, what a way to make a living;

Department of Health, it's all taking and no giving.

Alliance send you the wrong stuff and they never give you credit;

It's enough to drive you crazy, if you let it.

Six until four, the supermarket's got you where they want you;

There's a better life, and you dream about it, don't you?

It's a multiples game, no matter what they call it;

And you spend your life putting money in their wallet.

That Don't Impress Me Much

I've known a few guys who thought they were pretty
smart

But you've got being right down to an art

You think you're a genius-you drive me up the wall

You're a regular original, a know-it-all

Oh-oo-oh, you think you're special

Oh-oo-oh, you think you're something else

Okay, so you're a community pharmacist

That don't impress me much

So you got the blog but have you got the touch

Don't get me wrong, yeah I think you're alright

But that won't keep me warm in the middle of the night

That don't impress me much

I never knew a locum who carried a calculator in his
pocket

And a pen up his sleeve-just in case

And all those extra VAT petrol receipts in your wallet

'Cause Heaven forbid you should lose one

Oh-oo-oh, you think you're special

Oh-oo-oh, you think you're something else

Okay, so you're Mr Dispenser

That don't impress me much

So you got the words but have you got the touch

Don't get me wrong, yeah I think you're alright

But that won't keep me warm in the middle of the night

That don't impress me much

You're one of those guys who likes to shine his tablet counting machine

You make me wash my hands before you let use it

I can't believe you kiss your BNF good night

C'mon baby tell me-you must be jokin', right!

Oh-oo-oh, you think you're special

Oh-oo-oh, you think you're something else

Okay, so you've got a RP certificate

That don't impress me much

So you got the letters after your name but have you got
the touch

Don't get me wrong, yeah I think you're alright

But that won't keep me warm in the middle of the night

That don't impress me much

You think you're cool but have you got the touch

Don't get me wrong, yeah I think you're alright

But that won't keep me warm on the long, cold, lonely
night

That don't impress me much

Okay, so what do you think you're @MrDodgyChemist
or something...

Oo-Oh-Oh

That don't impress me much!

Oh-Oh-Oh-Oh-No

Alright! Alright!

You're Xrayser!

@pillmanuk maybe.

@aptaim.

Whatever!

That don't impress me much!

Christmas Song Lyrics about Pharmacy

1] Santa Claus is coming to town: *"He's making a list, And checking it twice; Gonna find out Who's naughty and nice"* = Is Santa a GPhC inspector?

2] Last Christmas: *"Last Christmas, I gave you my heart but the very next day, you gave it away"*= Clearly, this is about the time I gave Mrs Smith an emergency supply of Cardicor last Christmas and she promised she would start bringing in her prescriptions but she was lying!

3] Feed the World: *"Do they know it's Christmas time again?"* = NO, THEY BLOODY DON'T! TWO DAYS! TWO BLEEDING DAYS! THAT'S ALL WE ARE SHUT!... I'm ok now

4] All I want for Christmas: *"I don't want a lot for Christmas, There is just one thing I need"* = My 15 item prescription dispensing at 17.55pm on Xmas Eve...

5] Merry Xmas [War is Over]: *"Let's stop all the fight Now"* = GP receptionists and pharmacy staff should get on with each other

6] Fairytale of New York: *"They got cars big as bars /They got rivers of gold"* = GPs

7] Rudolph the red nose reindeer: *"Had a very shiny nose,/And if you ever saw it,/You would even say it glows."* = Does sir require a decongestant and some nose balm?

8] Step into Christmas: *"Welcome to my Christmas song/ I'd like to thank you for the year/ So I'm sending you this Christmas card /To say it's nice to have you here"* = Aw shucks but where is our tin of biscuits?!

GUEST BLOGS 1

Mr Dodgy Chemist

'Can I speak to the responsible pharmacist?' 'No. We don't have one.' 'How are you open then?' 'We just have a pharmacist.'

Shout out to pharmacies with USB ports so I can charge my phone and pretend to label at the same time.

Note to self - For future reference, when an annoyed patient asks you, *'You think you're a comedian?'* don't ask them if they're an agent.

Lady asked to have a word with the pharmacist and then walked off when she saw it was me. Really need to start displaying the right RP notice.

GPHC-*'What's your policy on confidential waste and it's destruction?' 'Only one person can use toilet at a time and must flush. Twice if needed.'*

'I've never had this drug before. Can you tell me why my doctor's prescribed it?' 'The drug rep is probably giving him commission.'

'Could you check and tell me if my Anusol suppositories are in?' 'It's not part of my job description to.

'I'm an Accredited Checking Technician so I can check too if you want.' 'Ok great could you check where my coffee's got to?'

You know you use Twitter too much when a patient asks you a question about their medicines and you check twitter for interactions and not the BNF.

*'This item is a special. It will be 2-3 working days.'
'What's so special about it?' 'Let's just say it makes us a lot of money.'*

'What is this 6 month gap on your CV?' 'I was suspended for not doing CPD.' 'You said that for the last gap.' 'Oh, I was in prison then.'

Calculations are key to passing the pre-reg exam. E.g. If your student debt is £20,000 and work available is 0, why did you waste your money?

'Would you be interested in our repeat collection service?' 'How does it work?' 'If you're too lazy to order it yourself, we do it for you.'

'These Orlistat pills are too big. Is there an easier way to swallow them?' 'Coat them in mayonnaise and they slide right in.'

People say there's no such thing as a free lunch but when you become a pharmacist there's no such thing as lunch.

'Your bread and crackers will be about 3-4 working days.' 'What am I supposed to do in the meantime?' 'Have an apple? Or a carrot?'

'Are you on any medication?' 'Just Methadone', I replied during the opening exchanges of my fitness to practice hearing.

Damn! I'm at the same store two days in a row. So got to iron a new shirt.

I base my emergency supply quantities on the amount of remaining tablets in the split pack.

I've just come up with a new weight loss pill. It's a placebo tablet which needs to be taken 8 times a day on an empty stomach.

'It takes about 3 working days which means from Mon...' 'Yes I know what a working day is.' 'But you tick K on your prescriptions?'

'Why isn't my prescription ready!?' 'The pharmacist got struck off while you were gone.'

'Why isn't my prescription ready?' 'I was hoping you wouldn't come back.'

'Have you had this before?' 'Yes, I have it pretty regularly,' I told the person chairing my Fitness To Practice hearing.

Awkward moment when you spend longer trying to find a shortcut for a direction than it would have been to just type it all out.

Why is it that every time I open a sealed box to take out a blister or two, I ALWAYS get the end with the PIL cuddling all the blisters?

If you get all the labels that are wasted in 1 year when you change a label roll and lay them out, you'd probably get fired for time wasting.

'Can I check, is this the first time you've had orlistat?'
'No, been on it for years.' 'Why haven't you lost weight then?'

If you spend two hours waiting at a walk-in centre for 24 Ibuprofen 400mg and 32 Paracetamol 500mg then you deserve all the pain in the world.

Why did the pharmacist cross the road? He was hungry and went to get a sandwich. Stop moaning you spoilt brats.

'Take TWO od for ONE week, ONE od for ONE week and then STOP.' Lady's been on these directions for two years now. I hope her day comes soon.

Patient once asked me why I always get his medications wrong. *'You see Mr Brown it's because...'* I started, *'It's Mr Hendry'* he interrupted.

"As directed" - The greatest 'pass the buck' in medical history.

Patient saw me getting my prescription at a rival pharmacy. Asked why not at my own pharm. I said I don't trust the pharmacist. 'That's you though..?'

Tumbleweed that rolls past when you ask patient to confirm address and they say different address, followed by the awkward handover.

Had patient with severe constipation. No bowel moment in 72 hours. Sent straight to hospital to maximise chances of catching Norovirus.

People often accuse Pharmacists of being wannabe Doctors. Or so my receptionist tells me. I don't deal much with the general public.

People often accuse pharmacists of being wannabe Doctors. Or so I'm told. I block out most noise with my stethoscope in my ears all day.

Awkward Moment when you finish speaking with a customer but they do not move or leave. You then realise they're waiting for a prescription.

A young lady just asked for my number! She was eager. She'd already taken it down from my RP notice before I even had a chance to apologise.

Xrayser

How come patients on JSA etc. are getting scripts for vitamin D? I stare at the sun through pharmacy window but they've time to lay out in it!

Our plasters currently offering "50% extra free" and customer has asked if he could just have the free 50% Oh how we laughed.

How can it take 2 minutes 47 seconds on the phone for a patient to effectively say "Please repeat my eight regular medicines?"

I had a supermarket pack of sushi for lunch yesterday. It is laid out in portions on a tray - it felt like I had an MDS pack for my food!

As there's a pregnancy test called "Answer", why don't we have a brand of condom called "Question"?

Every other script today has been for trimethoprim - there must be something in the water

Dashed next door for a breakfast roll - that was the idea of the Responsible Pharmacist regulations wasn't it?

I swear the pharmacy stamp has a cloak of invisibility around it.

Is it just me or does every pharmacist put something down then not find it? And then find it's on the bench in front of you.

Man just came in and said "We need some nit treatment." Jane: "How many are you treating?" Man: "Don't know - they're a bit too small to count."

Honestly. How do patients know which prescriptions you've checked (so don't collect for days) but always impatient for those buried at bottom of pile?

New product announcement - FORXIGA (dapagliflozin). Is this first drug with brand name more difficult to pronounce than the generic?

Patient just came in with a bad eye - because he tried to book an appointment with his surgery, and the system told him he doesn't exist!

Why do dispensers insist on cleaning PC equipment? - it always breaks it. Just had to re-assemble our client PC...

The stapler has legs - it keeps running away and hiding!

A lady on the counter used to work in local pub. She's great with customers and knows lots of people - but everyone she knows is on vitamin B.

Patient just told me she comes to us instead of our competitor because all his staff are so young. Not sure I take that as a compliment

Brief panic when I realised my left hand trouser pocket was empty! Now found my phone. Whatever did we have in our pockets before mobiles?

Large muscular tattooed bloke just bought Dioralyte as he's "dehydrated and got a fight in an hour" I assume for sport not healthy thuggery!

How difficult is it to work out amount of methadone to cover a Bank Holiday? Too difficult for our GPs. Why do FP10MDA prescriptions make their brains melt?

What do you give to the man who has everything? Antibiotics!

Just me, or does everyone have a dispenser who won't go to lunch on time because they think it's helpful to "just finish this" but then she's late back.

Ah - Autumn. Season of mists and staff complaints because half of them are too cold and the others too hot.

Bloke just came to pick up a prescription for his granddaughter - knew her first name but couldn't tell us her surname, address or date of birth.

Just had a bloke in the pharmacy hawking knocked-off mattresses. Is that what we've come to? Was tempted mind. - I fancy a kip.

What is it with patients and 'caplets' Do they insist their sandwiches are a particular shape? Is this the reason for chicken nuggets?

Just had pack of live maggot dressing delivered - all the girls want a look but disappointed you can't actually see the little blighters!

@weeneldo

Got a confession to make. All this time I've been making clarithromycin suspension with 40ml of water and not 39.9ml like the bottle says...

Was asked by patient "Does this cream have any chemicals in it?". WHAT DOES THAT EVEN MEAN?

Tip for men: If "the wife" sends you to the pharmacy, actually listen to what she asks you to buy because I can't work it out for you.

Pharmacists' children are the only kids who know the 28 times table before they learn any of the others.

Why are lollipops harder to open than medicine bottles?

Is it unethical and selfish that, as a locum, I kind of hope that other pharmacists get the winter vomiting bug and can't come to work?

When I was at university we were filmed doing OTC. Wasn't realistic though, no one asked for 32 Solpadeine Plus.

You should have a TV show about your sales techniques: The Only Way is Ethics.

Or a South African version called Cash in the Ethic.

The first time I tried to demonstrate a Nicorette Quickmist I went in unprepared...ended up with 3 dead, 15 injured.

If ever there was a candidate for Ritalin, it's Norman from Fireman Sam. It's a miracle he hasn't burnt Pontypandy to the ground yet.

Ever shout a patient's name then feel like a total dick when you realise no-one is in the shop?

I love when the phone goes and an unspoken tension rapidly builds in the room as you all wait for someone else to answer.

Levothyroxine? L? E? Nope, T for thyroxine! Warfarin at W except 0.5mg at M. Isosorbide Mononitrate in like nine different places.

I had a guy's prescription, all prime numbers: 149 Baclofen, 31 Ramipril etc. Every month since forever.

The more embarrassed you look when getting Viagra/condoms, the more we'll talk about you when you leave.

Got a friend on JSA? Want free scripts? Just say you went out right before you signed the prescription and split up right after. Sorted.

I had a dental script for erythromycin TDS. Told dentist usually QDS he said "I never realised, I just always do antibiotics TDS"

Worst thing ever is getting a new prescription on a Saturday with "as directed" and brought in by the patient's next door neighbour.

I hate how difficult it is to Google pharmacy stuff without getting 'Canadian Viagra pharmacy online cheap buy' for half the results.

I worked at one of the big chains recently; apparently some guy called FRED has a weird fetish for velcroing staplers to the wall.

All the extemporaneous knowledge needed: Add teabag to mug. Add boiling water to fill mug. Remove bag. Add sugar and milk to taste.

During university, I imagined one day having my certificate, how proud I'd feel. Qualified 2011, they stopped certificates! Gutted!

Locum blues: Crazy Sat, me and one counter assistant, no time to write up/pour meth Locum joy: I don't have to sort it on Monday.

I am such a hypocrite. Got antibiotics the other day and have been failing miserably at taking them. I'm part of the problem.

A question for anyone working in pharmacy: have you ever been in a shop that's a good temperature? It's always either frostbite or heatstroke.

I can't wait to be old. I'll be a BASTARD. I'll want specific drug brands, get deliveries but be out, I'll have earned it!

'Are you on any medication?' 'No, just the pill and inhalers.' Can someone explain? I was off ill when they explained Yes and No at Uni.

It's your fault by Becky Morley

Tucked out of the way in an office working as a pharmacy technician at the local GP practice, I was having a quiet morning drinking my much needed coffee while looking at prescribing data, when the phone rang.

It was one of the practice receptionists, in her usual pleasant calm manner she said *'I have a lady here who has a problem with her prescription, I wondered if you would be able to help her?'* *'What is the problem? Does it need the GP or can I help?'* I replied. *'You should be able to help her. I have asked her to take a seat in the waiting area'* the receptionist said. *'Ok, I will go through'* I put the phone down, picked up my note pad and pen and headed towards the waiting area.

Patients often came in with queries, such as, 'these look different to last time' or that they have been taking too many so have ran out sooner than expected and need more, so I was used to dealing with these problems. The practice seemed quiet on the way to the waiting area, no babies screaming, people coughing or even the mumble of the oldies having a social chat discussing ailments while waiting for the doctor.

It all became clear as soon as I entered the waiting area. I knew straight away who I had been asked to help. I wanted to turn and run back to the safety of my office, but it was too late, I had been seen. This was no lady. Rising on hind legs as I approached was a double-headed, fire breathing dragon expelling steam from its ears, my presence seemed to fuel the anger from within. Striding towards me, baring teeth she extended her arm to point a long bony finger in my chest.

'WHY IS MY PRESCRIPTION NOT AT THE PHARMACY? I HAVEN'T HAD MY MORNING TABLET. I DEMAND TO KNOW. IT'S YOUR FAULT...' I was aware all eyes in the waiting room were on me; no one dare breathe or move a muscle. I was ridged with fear, couldn't speak and out of the corner of my eye I could see the 'zero tolerance to staff' poster but couldn't even raise my arm to point at it. I slowly stepped back, she plunged 'ARE YOU LISTENING TO ME? ARE YOU? WHAT ARE YOU GOING TO DO?' I was silent, for what seemed like an eternity, willing myself to speak.

With shaking hands I lifted the pad and paper, she held my gaze. 'Sorry about that. Can you please write your name and date of birth on here for me along with the medication you are looking for and I will go and check if the doctor has processed the prescription' The pad and pen was snatched from my hand, she let out a grunt as she started to scratch on to my note pad her details. The patients were all still looking at me as if to say 'fancy showing yourself up like that' but not one of them daring to say it. The note pad was thrust back into my hand while she was still double, no, triple underlining the details. I asked her to take a seat and told her I would be as quick as possible and go straight to the GP.

I turned and with my head down scurried off down the corridor back to my desk, heart pounding, holding back tears - after all, we don't have training to deal with aggression while doing the Tech course at college. I got to my office closed the door, took a deep breath to compose myself, as I would probably have to go and speak to the doctor. I looked down at my note pad, under the name and date of birth, etched in to my note pad said 'HRT!' I smiled to myself, it explained a lot.

I checked the computer, issued the prescription and got it signed by the GP. It was time to come face to face again, at least this time I had what she wanted, maybe this encounter wouldn't be as bad, surely? I cautiously walked towards her, stretched out my arm holding the prescription, not daring to make eye contact 'sorry about th...' I started to speak but I couldn't finish. She burst into tears, thanked me profusely for all my help and headed off. I noticed the waiting room in stunned silence. I hoped that they all don't try and pull this off when their prescription isn't at the pharmacy on time!

John D'Arcy

I was once part of a meeting of pharmacy luminaries and we were debating some issue (its nature now escapes me but at the time there was no doubt in our minds that it was one that was fundamental to our professional future.) It was so important that the Chairman insisted no one could leave the room until we had a resolution to the problem and insisted that everyone turn phones off to avoid all distractions. The meeting had been going on in earnest for around one hour when a phone started ringing. Everyone at the meeting started tutting and looking around in disgust. Meanwhile, the culprit grabbed his phone and apologised saying this was an important business call he had to take, and to the chagrin of all, particularly the chairman, he left the room.

Upon his departure there ensued a discussion around how wrong it was that this individual had left his phone on and how disruptive this was to the intensive debate we were having. Seconds later, the door swung open with such force that it nearly parted company with its hinges. The guy who had taken the phone call stood there with his phone at his ear holding the door open. He bellowed to the group.

"Thyroxine is increasing in price by 70% tomorrow afternoon".

87

There was no comment from anybody. Instead, they got up and left the room (at a pace that would have given Usain Bolt some difficulty) grabbing hold of their mobiles as they went. You knew that within five minutes there would be no thyroxine stock left in circulation.

A matter of principle

I attended an LPC meeting once and one of the main topics on the agenda was a proposal by the Department of Health that pharmacists check prescription exemptions as a means of clumping down on patients making incorrect claims. This was a sensitive issue for the profession. Historically, pharmacists had never countenanced such a role on the basis that such a role would come between the delicate pharmacist/patient relationship that was founded in large part on trust and confidence. So, the tone of the meeting was resolutely in favour of saying "no" to such an outrageous proposal.

After considerable debate – with virtually everyone being in favour of saying "no" – the Chairman summed up. He said,

"This is a very simple issue. From an LPC perspective, we need to consider what our members would want us to do. They would not want us selling them down the river by agreeing to this nonsensical proposal that would see pharmacists becoming exemption policemen and the enemy of our patients. This is a matter of absolute

principle that goes to the foundation of our professional status", he said, We must say no"

At the meeting was a PSNC Regional Representative who came back at the Chairman,

"What if there was money involved?" he said

"That would depend on how much?" said the Chairman.

Shipman Inquiry

I gave evidence at the Shipman Inquiry. On the way to the Inquiry the solicitor who accompanied me asked what I wanted to get out of the process. I said that there were two things I wanted to achieve; firstly to make sure pharmacy's voice was heard so that we did not become the scapegoat of the Inquiry; secondly to tell the Chairman of the Inquiry, Dame Janet Smith, a joke. The solicitor looked alarmed at the second objective.

"You cannot tell a High Court Judge a joke" he said, "particularly during the course of a high profile public inquiry such as this. Besides it will look terrible in the transcript".

"Relax", I said, "I was only kidding".

During the course of the Inquiry we got into a rather technical discussion around the legality of supplying POMs and CDs and as part of this a difference of opinion emerged where we were arguing that a particular set of circumstances amounted to an offence of supply. The Department of Health disagreed with this suggesting that no such offence would exist. I held my ground and argued back that there would be an offence of supply. Dame Janet looked at me and said,

"So you mean to tell me that if I took my husband's prescription only medicines, I would be guilty of an offence of supply?"

In reply I said,

"If you did this Dame Smith I suggest you would be guilty of an offence of theft."

The room erupted in laughter. Objective two achieved!

MY BLOGS 2

Taking in a prescription

Amusing when you ask patients to sign the prescription and they sign next to the doctors signature.

Britain has a problem. No one likes to read. I know this because no one carries their reading glasses when they have to sign a prescription!

The 'Evidence not seen' box on a prescription is powerful when you use it.

Why do some people not sit down until you ask them and others sit down when you want them to stand up and pay for their prescription?

When people start getting grumpy at our waiting times, I like to do a Fire Drill.

The most dangerous thing in pharmacy is two old people discussing the waiting time loudly. Very loudly. This is how revolutions start.

Our waiting time was so long today that the lady waiting for her zolpidem started yawning

Whenever I get my own prescription dispensed, I take it into a pharmacy two minutes before they shut. They always do it super quick and even hold the door open for me on the way out.

Patient: *'How much?!?! It was £5.90 the last time I got a prescription!'* Me:*' Congratulations on being healthy the last 10 years.'*

£7.85 in copper coins?!?! Have you been saving up for this Chlamydia treatment?

So, you aren't happy with our 10mins waiting time and would rather go to the pharmacy 10mins away? Ok then.

Annoying moment when counter assistant takes the actual waiting time and divides it by ten and gives patient the answer.

Patient today: *'Can you hurry as I'm off to play golf and am already late?'*

Exemption

It annoys me when patients double-tick the back of their script. That's just greedy! It makes me chuckle when people tick income support on their baby's prescription. The parents fill in the prescription but write down their exemption instead of the child's.

Students start university at 18 years of age and get quite upset when they hit 19 and realise that they have to pay. I have seen students blatantly lie about their age even though it is printed on the prescription.

Pharmacy staff members sometimes fill out the back of the prescription for people who are exempt by age, when we receive the prescription from the doctor's. Sometimes, they tick over 60 when the patient is not. One day, I will get a slap when handing out a prescription for an insecure 55 year old lady.

There is no requirement for someone over 60 to sign the back of their prescription if it is a printed prescription as it's obvious from the date of birth that they will be exempt. Depending on how grumpy the person is, I do or do not make them sign.

Sometimes, you may ask someone to pay and they say that they are over 60 and it's confirmed by looking at the prescription properly. If you apologise and say that they look good for their age, then you will get brownie points.

Sometimes, pregnant ladies will ask me if I want to see their exemption card but I say that I can see their evidence. This is either a big bump or a baby. Sometimes, maternity exemption is ticked by a man with medical exemption by accident which causes much hilarity and embarrassment for the man.

People with certain conditions get free prescriptions. These include epilepsy, diabetes and under active thyroid. Recently, cancer was added to the list which is excellent. However, my Auntie was over the moon when she got diabetes as she now has free prescriptions for life.

Unfortunately, some people don't believe that the prepayment certificate is a good offer. I once wasted 5mins of my life explaining the benefits of a pre-payment complete with calculations and my working out and they couldn't be bothered. I'm more upset about having to do some calculations. The prepayment certificate also encourages people to be ill [or lie and pretend to be ill] to make it cost-effective.

Some women who have another non-contraceptive item on the prescription, sometimes conveniently forget to pay for that item and just tick X. These women get chased after by overweight pharmacists.

A guy came in with a T-Shirt that said 'Guess' on it. I asked, "Income support?" Some people who can't speak English just say 'H' when asked what they tick. It is also normally ticked by people in expensive cars who have just come back from holidaying abroad. Jobseekers allowance is normally ticked by people in McDonald's uniform and taxi drivers.

'Do you pay for your prescription?'

'No, I have a white card'

'Which one?'

'Dunno'

It wasn't me

I want to share with you some of the excuses I have heard from staff when they make a dispensing near miss. I appreciate that we are all human and, therefore, make mistakes but I can't help feeling annoyed when instead of a simple apology and moment of recognition the following excuses are blurted out on a daily basis as to why the mistake occurred:

1] It is too hot

2] It is too cold

3] I am hungry

4]. I had too much to eat at lunch

5] It wasn't me (no one owns up and the label is not signed)

6] It wasn't me (they dispute it even though they have signed the label)

7] I just stuck the labels on, I did not dispense it

8] The box is a different colour and I got confused

9] The box is the same colour; it's just a different drug unfortunately

10] I labelled it as amoxicillin 500mg so don't understand why the label came out as amoxicillin 250mg

11] I'm thirsty

12] I need a wee

13] That's what they had last time

14] I didn't label it, it's the labeller's fault

15] I thought it said glycerin suppositories not glyceryl trinitrate spray. Is there a difference?

Deliveries

Nowadays, if you don't offer a delivery service then you are losing customers. People expect a delivery service.

It used to be that only housebound patients were eligible for delivery. The rules have changed now. The 100-hour pharmacy down the road started offering it to anyone and now we have to do the same.

It is quite annoying when lazy jobless (but capable of work) people ask for deliveries. They can manage to drive to the shops to pick up cigarettes and alcohol but are unable to pick up their Champix and Campral themselves.

And then you have the 'Demanders'. These people want to know exactly what time the delivery will arrive so they don't miss any of Jeremy Kyle. Others are perfectly happy for you to push it through the letterbox. They don't understand that we need a signature. Most things that get delivered need a signature these days except takeaways. Ah, I see now why they get confused!

And then you have the urgent deliveries that always seem to be life and death. *'The surgery are faxing it over'* they say. When the fax arrives, the Gaviscon or paracetamol on it makes my BP rise steeply!

Don't get me wrong. I would do anything to help my patients. I have frequently delivered medicines after work, on foot, even in the snow. Just don't make me come and let me see your car in the driveway!

If you keep asking for your medication to be delivered and posted through the letter box, I'll start popping them through one by one.

Day Off

I wake up at 7am automatically and can't get back to sleep.

Make a cup of coffee at 9am and finish it at 11am

On the toilet when the delivery driver calls.

Ring company to ask driver to attempt re-delivery.

Driver comes again when I have nipped out to fish and chip shop.

Driver shouts at me for not being in and says that I shouldn't have lunch.

Neighbour calls round to borrow some paracetamol as she has run out.

Friend sends me a picture of his Haemorrhoids and wants me to recommend something. I recommend a new friend.

Dad rings me to ask about the latest Daily Mail Cancer scare story.

I ring the surgery and want a quick word with my GP but am told she is busy.

I want to do a crossword but can't find a pen.

I get a phone call about PPIs. Decide to give the caller a lecture about how lansoprazole works.

Mum rings me on my landline to ask if I am home.

A rep knocks on the door and wants to talk to me about double glazing but I won't let him in.

The kids won't listen to me or do as they are told. They frequently answer back.

They make a cake for their grandparents but end up using salt instead of sugar. It was a serious baking error.

I have to apologise to my angry in-laws and make the kids write a letter of apology.

I always look forward to a day off from the pharmacy.

Awkward pharmacy moments

When you can't read your own handwriting. How do doctors cope?!?

When the till roll starts going red and you calmly walk away and hope someone else changes it...

When a dispenser tries to dispense someone 100mg of Viagra instead of 25mg and you wonder if they are going out secretly.

When the person that talks the most at work, complains about someone else that talks too much...

When you are in the middle of a serious conversation and the other person's stomach grumbles and you have to pretend not to notice.

On a Friday when you tell a patient to call back for an owing the next day and then remember when they are gone that you are shut on Saturdays.

When you get a patient to fill out a patient satisfaction questionnaire and then have to tell them a minute later about an owing.

When you turn around in the dispensary and there is a little old lady standing right behind you and you scream!

When a patient asks you a question about a disease that only Dr House is aware of and you slip away and Google it.

When you realise a patient has not paid and they have left. Silence as all staff stare at each other deciding who has to run.

When you locum on the weekend and you don't want your company to find out and you spot your area manager!

Fussy Patients

Don't you just hate fussy patients? Every pharmacy has them. People who want a specific generic. Mrs P wants white atenolol as the orange gives her diarrhoea. Mr S wants orange atenolol as the white gives him constipation. Mr T can only have Bristol Metformin because the others taste funny while Mrs X will die if she does not get Actavis Prednisolone.

You try to explain in vain that it's the same medication, just made by somebody else, but they never listen. Sometimes it is easy enough. You just have to pick a different box off the shelf. Most times it's not that easy. You have to ring your wholesaler to ask for the specific generic. It is generally more expensive than the generic that you normally keep in. Sometimes you ask for a white tablet and then get sent five different generics in the hope that one is white.

You have to add a note to the patients PMR to remind you that they like a specific generic. Then you have to add another note to remind you not to ignore the first note. You don't get a specific thank you every time you get the specific generic for the patient but you do get a bollocking if you don't. This generally happens when you have a locum who is not familiar with their needs.

Dispensersize

DO YOU WORK IN PHARMACY?

DO YOU LIKE CAKES?

Then this work-out video is for YOU

I guarantee that you will lose pounds! 39.99 to be exact!

1] Encourage people to not pay for their prescription. Give them a 30 second head start and then run after them. Great for cardio.

2] Stretch for those items on the top shelf.

3] Keep making near-misses when dispensing so you have to walk back and forth to the pharmacist. A great way to increase your steps.

4] If short, stand on your tiptoes so you can see over the counter. Great for your calves.

5] Engage in NMS: No More Sugar.

6] Do more MURS: Motivate Urself Really Severely.

7] Step aerobics using the kick stool.

8] Popping tablets makes your fingers stronger.

POP CULTURE 2

Apprentice Pharmacy Cliches

The clichés used on the Apprentice can be used in the pharmacy:

1] *"I like to think outside the box"* = I stick the label outside the box that says 'Affix label'

2] *"I give 110%"* = I give 30 fluoxetine instead of the prescribed 28

3] *"I have a proven track record in sales"* = I sell co-codamol to anybody

4] *"I stepped up"* = I used the kick stool

5] *"I'm passionate"* = I love pens

6] *"There are no friends in business"* = My staff members hate me

7] *"It was your/her/his/responsibility"* = Who forgot to order paracetamol?

8] *"Why have you brought x back into the boardroom?"* = Why are you doing an MUR on antibiotics for Mrs Smith?

9] *"I've left (blank) behind to come here"* = I used to be a manager at KFC, now I want to be an area manager for your multiple

Celebrity Service

We have had several famous people attend our pharmacy to use our services.

Don Draper from Mad Men attends our smoking cessation service. He is failing miserably.

Norm from Cheers comes in to the Alcohol screening service and everybody knows his name in the pharmacy.

Renton from Trainspotting comes in daily for his methadone.

Christian Grey accessed the Chlamydia screening service on several occasions.

Monica from Friends lost her excess baggage by using our Weight Management Service.

The Waltons came in for Minor Ailments when one of them got Threadworm.

And Barney from How I Met Your Mother got some Viagra using our PGD.

Songs about Pharmacy

1] Hot Chocolate: *It Started With A Kiss* - Why do you need EHC?

2] Paloma Faith: *Picking Up The Pieces* - Smashed Conical

3] Annie Lennox: *Walking on Broken Glass* - Smashed Conical 2

4] Elvis: *A Little Less Conversation* - All staff

5] The Weather Girls: *It's Raining Men* - Senior positions in pharmacy organisations

6] Natalie Imbruglia: *Torn* - Tearing the repeat slip

7] Backstreet Boys: *As Long As You Love Me* - Bending over backwards for a patient

8] Take That: *Back for Good* - Recurrent Candida

9] Kelly Clarkson: *Mr Know-It-All* - Annoying pharmacist with a clinical diploma

10] Tiffany: *I Think We're Alone Now* - Private word with the pharmacist

Monologues and theme tunes

A-Team

In 2002, Frank 'Hannibal' Dispenser was disciplined by a multiple for a dispensing error he didn't commit. He promptly ignored the letter and moved to Yorkshire. Today, still wanted by the NHS, he survives as locum of fortune. If you have a shift that needs covering- if no one else can help - and if you can find him and pay mileage, then - maybe you can hire: Mr D

Hannibal sometimes works with a tech with bad attitude called Barbara Baracus, a good looking delivery driver called Tina 'The Face' Peck and a howling mad counter assistant called Mandy Murdock.

@DrChrisGreen: Is the local GPhC inspecter Colonel Decker (retired)?

Dirty Harry

I know what you're thinking: "Did he count five tablets or only four?" Well, to tell you the truth, in all this excitement I kinda lost track myself.

But as this is a treatment for bacterial vaginosis – the most powerful disease down below in the world and one that could blow your area clean off – you've got to ask yourself one question: "Do I feel lucky?" Well, do ya, miss?

Taken

I don't know who you are. I don't know what you want. If you are looking for ransom, I can tell you I don't have money due to the global recession and category M.

But what I do have is a very particular set of skills – skills I have acquired over summer vacation placements, four years of university and one year's training. Skills that make me a nightmare for doctors.

If you let my pen go now, that'll be the end of it. I will not look for you, I will not pursue you. But if you don't, I will look for you, I will find you and I will kill you.

Mrs Doubtfire

Anybody remember the film Mrs Doubtfire? You know, the one in which Frank Dispenser gets fired as a pharmacist manager and dresses up as an old Scottish lady pharmacist and comes back as the new manager in disguise and has pretend hot flushes?

Patient Confidentiality

[amended scene from Austin Powers: International Man of Mystery]

Austin Powers is chatting up the young counter assistant. Mr Dispenser appears.

Mr Dispenser: *'One Swedish-made penis pump for Mr Powers'*

Austin Powers: [to the counter assistant] *'That's not mine'*

Mr Dispenser: *'One credit card receipt for Swedish-made penis pump signed by Austin Powers'*

Austin Powers: *'I'm telling ya baby, that's not mine'*

Mr Dispenser: *'One NHS receipt for penis pump, filled out for Austin Powers so you can claim it back'*

Austin Powers: *'I don't even know what this is! This sort of thing is a one-off. Never to be repeated'*

Mr Dispenser: *'One repeat slip for Austin Powers for penis pump so you can order it again'*

SOCIAL MEDIA 2

Outside the Pharmacy

I always panic when some people try and park outside the pharmacy as they only leave one inch between the car and us. What's the strangest thing you have seen happen outside your pharmacy?

1] @brennanpharm: Elephant

2] @kim_whitehouse: A scene from a movie being filmed! It was called 'Goal'

3] @eoin_martin: Patient turns up for daily prescription with an eagle on their arm...

4] @RPHTOTHESTARS: A couple, 70 year plus getting it on by the store's dumpster.

5] @Rose_Amos: A man walking by dressed as a hotdog.

6] @Doriannjb: I had a woman come in for self-tan, she realised she needed to shave her legs, she bought a razor, sat, and shaved her legs.

7] @i_Q_Balls: A brawl. It was pretty funny as they both ticked box 'C' on the prescription.

8] @Gordon1000: A policeman chasing a suspect who escaped through a plate glass window from inside a shop on the other side of the road.

9] @__shell: Patient takes time to wait on his bag of meds and then walks across the road, takes out an inhaler and dumps rest in bin.

10] @JanetTozer: Patient arrived to collect prescription in an army tank.

11] Billy B: When I was in Australia I worked at a beachside pharmacy in Shoal Bay. I once saw a huge kangaroo hop along the main road right outside our pharmacy! Quick those things.

Being Late

What's the funniest excuse that you have heard someone give for being late to work?

1] Ronnie P: *"Sorry I was late, I had to go to the Pharmacy to collect my prescription"*

2] @CheekyBandari: My area manager rang before I arrived so when I returned his call and got a grilling as to why I was late, my response was:

"Bowel problems"

He left it at that. This also works with:

"Period problems" too.

3] Corinne M: *"I wasn't late I've been sat in the car park the last 15mins, waiting for the rain to stop!"* It didn't stop, it got heavier.

4] Si B: *"I was late leaving the gym and stopped off at McDonald's on way here!"*

5] Heather P: A friend of mine was late once because she got stuck in a lift.

6] Sabina R: *"Sorry I'm late I missed my alarm. My 8 month old son must have woken up in the night and turned it off."*

7] Khalil A: *"I left the shop keys at home and only realised when I got to the shop. I had to drive back home. As the keys were in the coat I wore yesterday!"*

8] Clarice S: (From a guy) It was raining and he had to go back home and do his hair again

9] Lynn P: *"Sorry I am late (again).I was picking apples off my tree for you all!"*

10] Gina E: I'm late? No, must be your watch.

11] Nicki P: One guy said he was late because his girlfriend wouldn't let him get out of bed because he was too good looking - too much information!

12] Sharon R: *"My brother came in for the nightshift late, saying he'd fallen off his skateboard on the way to work. He's nearly 40."*

13] Jill T: *"Sorry I was late, the bus driver made me finish my coffee before he would let me get on the bus!"*

14] Adam P: *"I thought I was late but then my period started thank God."* Crossed wires I suppose, but it was a good response!

15] Nikki Jane S: "My car wouldn't start" They lived within 10 minutes walking distance.

16] @PhlyingRPh: I had an employee who "forgot to put the clocks back" an hour the last Sunday in October and was late on Monday

17] @dakafub: "My windscreen was frozen over." I should point out he was my second pharmacist but he was three hours late.

18] @frandavi99: *"I got arrested."*

19] @AngharadBond: *"I fell off the toilet and got a concussion, had to rescue a cow and my hubby put Baileys in my cocoa so I slept until 12pm and now there is no point in coming in really."* These were all from the same person too!

20] @Pharm_Thoughts *"I was stuck in the McDonald's drive thru."*

Awkward dispensing moments

1] @MrDispenser: Awkward moment when you dispense a script for someone that you went to school with and you wait to see whether they acknowledge you or not.

2] @JoMyatt: I had that on Thursday. I told him he was the year above me and he knew me! Clearly, I've not changed in 20 years.

3] Arlene C: Even better when it's a teacher who taught you at school!

4] @MrHunnybun: Very true, I can never tell if they genuinely don't remember me or are pretending not to because they have a prescription for 1g of Azithromycin.

5] @Raman2089: I had a prescription for an old teacher once. I was so tempted to ask him but decided against it!

6] @alkemist1912: Particularly when their prescription is for something like Methadone or maybe for an STD. I've had to deal with both situations.

7] @Alkemist1912: Or that awkward EHC for someone's wife/partner - and you know that they're supposed to be home alone!

8] @Andychristo: Been there! Awkward moment, especially as it was for a stat dose of Azithromycin.

9] @Checkedshoes: EHC with friend of daughter.

10] @Kevfrost: Even more awkward when you present an FP10 and see it's someone you trained in pharmacy.

11] @gemmieangel: Or when old geography teacher wants advice about the failure of his 'privates' when he has important lady friend to impress!

Wholesalers

@Lucycaulfield: Wholesaler left a Stanley knife in one of our delivery boxes. I didn't order this.

@AdamPlum: Item received Bard catheter tray: Item ordered diltiazem 60mr tabs.

@rikash_p: FedEx driver set the bar by giving a large stock order to a household because we were shut, didn't see him again.

@JemimaMcC: I can't relax until the totes are stacked with big totes on the bottom and little totes inside and lids on top.

@KirstyFM: I like mixing up how I stack the tote boxes, gives the AAH guys something to play with! Alliance ones make good storage boxes!

Neelm S: The best box is one with a piece of paper telling you that you have exceeded quota on all the items you ordered for owings!

@MrDispenser: I like seeing wholesaler vans driving around and wondering which pharmacy they are running late to get to next.

@MrDispenser: I watch too many spy films. Every time we have a different wholesaler driver, I fear for Bill's safety and think someone is trying to steal my book.

Aisha A: Wholesaler drivers have a real problem in picking up totes. Morning driver doesn't want to pick up evening ones and evening driver doesn't want to pick up morning ones.

Clauds D: This one woman stores all the goods down her top. Then takes them out to give them to you.

@LouiseAliceX: Wholesaler driver in Birmingham said to me that he was in Emmerdale as an extra. It's his claim to fame.

@bianca1319: We're very lucky, have great drivers. One has brought in homemade food and taught me a little salsa in the dispensary!

@ZainyBebe: I heard some were having affairs with the dispensers!

@theancientartof: One of our wholesaler drivers is the son of a pharmacist which makes him really understanding of our needs.

@brendansemple One of our delivery drivers played for Celtic in a European Cup Semi-final.

@Uninspirational: Our driver is always cheery. He even joined in our secret Santa at Christmas.

@Sarayummymummy: My driver even opens our boxes up and everything. Mind you I bribe them with cakes!

@helenroot: Mine were always lovely but I find being a massive flirt with them helps.

@jadewatt: Once asked our driver "oh what have you brought us today" and got the response "Argg its pirate treasure" (accent included).

@brendansemple: There's another driver who was in the GB Karate team who won the World Championship.

@MrDispenser: Dear wholesaler, think of a box of drugs as a shopping bag and the invoice as a tray of eggs. Don't put the invoice at the bottom of the box.

@MrDispenser: Awkward moment when AAH are late and you start to wonder whether you actually sent the order yesterday.

@MrDispenser: Remember the good old days when you could sign for an AAH delivery without having to have a degree in Computer Science.

@Xrayser: Ah - the wholesaler lottery. Order one enforced outer and they break them and send a single. But sometimes we order one and get an outer!

@Xrayser: How is it that when our wholesaler driver changes, the arrival time varies by up to an hour? Do some of them have a secret shortcut?

@Xrayser: Why do main wholesaler drivers have to come in pairs on a Saturday?

For Sale

Pharmacists are professionals. We are NOT shopkeepers. We would never sell ridiculous items in the pharmacy. What is the stupidest thing that you have seen for sale in a pharmacy?

1] Carley E: JLS condoms.

2] Lorna-Jane D: Paternity tests.

3] Steve T: Shoelaces, home brew kits and accessories, wool, knitting needles, patterns etc.

4] Hiba A: A beauty chair with a woman threading women's eye brows while waiting for their scripts.

5] Melissa B: Glass angels, made nice tree decorations though.

6] Bianca W: Coffee/tea flask.

7] Genevieve C: China tea sets.

8] Rachel G: Chocolate. I mean come on chocolate! There's your metformin sir and the 5 Mars bars!

9] Molly-Anne P: Squash? Socks?

10] Stuart H: Bloody photo kiosks that never work properly.

11] Helen R: Brewing kits were always sold in pharmacy in the days that pharmacists were 'chemists' and understood chemistry! Brewing is an arm of chemistry! I remember so much fab stuff being sold in pharmacies. We're hung up on the 'clinical pharmacy' these days and have lost the 'community' part that made us a part of it. The crazy stuff got people in our pharmacies and everyone went to the 'chemist'! I remember as a Saturday girl weighing out and bagging up dried fruit and nuts, labelled with dispensary printed labels!! Shock horror. Loved it.

12] Sarah P: Eggs! And there was an out-of-hours place that doubled as on off-licence. Two counters.

13] Joanne 'O'R: I used to work in pharmacy and at one time we used to sell espadrilles and plastic jelly shoes.

14] Rani R: Slippers and cardigans?

15] AZ M: Ammunition.

16] Julie G: I did an acquisition about 9 years ago and the stockroom has 1200 Beanie babies inside.

17] Meesha C: Scotch eggs, Witches tights and home tattoo kits.

18] Thomas V: Individual scrabble pieces.

19] @lifeonthepharm: Copper bracelet for realigning the body's energy fields.

20] @andychristo: Don't know about stupid, but oddest thing was fuse wire. Not fuses but actual fuse wire.

21] @oisinohalmhain: A lot of stuff in Irish retail pharmacies, especially multiples: George Foreman grill, stereo, hat boxes, silverware, chess set

22] @Theancientartof: Spirits, wine and cigarettes in a Welsh pharmacy in 70's - it was the only shop in the village!

23] @Mexican_Badger: Vajazzle. No joke.

24] @phuriouspharmer : Inflatable kiddy-size dinghy.

25] @AdamPlum: Mugs, £1 turkey roasting trays, paint rollers, paint brushes.

26] @CodeRedShell: Glow in the dark dog collar and lead.

27] @himalmakwana: Toy cars. It was the only reason I went into the pharmacy as a kid with my mum.

28] @Rachairley: Cigarettes! I lived in the US!

29] @Cleverestcookie: Vacuum cleaner.

20 Reasons why you can't sleep

1] @Genty_Rocks: Just finished my shift at 11pm and am back at 7am.

2] @MrDispenser: You bought 5000 boxes of simvastatin 40mg and then the surgery decided to listen to MHRA guidance for a change.

3] @googlybear84: It's your turn to open up and you haven't been given any keys.

4] @MrDispenser: Your superintendent/boss is following you on Twitter.

5] @Cleverestcookie: You took your furosemide at 6pm.

6] @MrDispenser: You forgot to send the order.

7] @shn86: You forgot your WWHAM questions when selling a box of paracetamol

8] @Cleverestcookie: You've just woken from a nightmare in which someone was cutting up calendar packs.

9] @shn86: Your locum was a right fittie and you turned up to work looking like a tramp.

10] @MrDispenser: That angry old lady is coming in tomorrow and Vagifem is on quota.

11] @sheeba_x: You left a controlled drug on the checking bench!

12] @Cleverestcookie: Because tomorrow is Monday and you're excited about working again.

13] @Cleverestcookie: You're locuming at the busy supervised methadone pharmacy where all the clients are related and look similar.

14] @Cleverestcookie: You're locuming at that pharmacy again with no staff, aggressive customers and poor stock control.

15] @Cleverestcookie: Just remembered that you promised to deliver a prescription on the way home and it's still on the bench.

16] @EmilyJaneBond82: Too busy making voodoo dolls of the pharma reps that pester you when you're trying to eat your lunch.

17] @MrDispenser: Stupid PCT pharmacist convinced the GP to stop prescribing me zopiclone.

18] @MrDispenser: That angry old man is coming in the morning and Cialis is on quota.

19] @MrDispenser: You ran out of methadone and so used washing up liquid. Addicts did not notice.

20] @MrDispenser: You haven't met your weekly MUR target of 100.

GUEST BLOGS 2

Pharm and Farm: A comparison by @lifeonthepharm

I have come to realise a similarity, other than pronunciation, of the Farming industry and Pharmacy.

1] Both often have to deal with rather large, uncooperative charges and both the farmer and Pharmacist have to come to deduce meaning from incomprehensible grunts.

2] Bad smells are part of daily duties, the majority from our respective herds.

3] Long hours are a common occurrence with the Locum and 100 hour pharmacist often rising early with the farmer and working late beyond nightfall.

4] Heavy lifting is a characteristic usually associated with the outdoors profession but I have encountered totes containing drinks which could easily slip a disc.

5] On a more serious note, both professions are facing squeezing of reimbursements.

6] .and diversification of business is one way to stay in the black whether this is through farm shops, ice-cream and cheese, or through MURs, NMS and EHC.

7] In modern times both sectors are facing ever increasing bureaucracy and paperwork, putting a squeeze on that most valuable resource: time.

8] The overuse of medicine seems to be an issue solely centred on healthcare, but the overuse of antibiotics in animals is a problem which is front and centre in many people's minds.

9] A degree of autonomy is a shared characteristic, with the treating of minor ailments dealt with internally within our respective fields, although we often have to answer to a higher power whether this is the supermarkets (which profession?) or targets from head office.

10] I'm sure many pharmacists have been asked to look into their crystal ball to answer those unanswerable questions (how long will I have the squits? When can I stop my citalopram?) and I have heard farmers being called upon themselves (is it going to be a hot summer? When should I pick my strawberries from the garden?)

11] Last but not least, the universal trait among Pharmacists and Farmers is the ability to deal with huge amounts of bullshit and keep going every day.

Pharmacist's Guide to Speed Dating by Helen Root

I enjoy a good conversation on Twitter and I have to say I have met some lovely new Pharmacy friends on there. However, I can't help thinking some days that we Pharmacists are strange individuals at times. Maybe strange is unfair, maybe I should say passionate or inquisitive. No, I'll stick with strange.

We get into arguments with a person we've never met, about which of us works the hardest, is the cleverest, is the most professional, the list goes on. What happens when you mix these strange creatures called Pharmacists in a room? And here was born

"The Pharmacists' guide to Speed Dating". Those 6 must ask questions that could change your life forever.

Now, before those of you Pharmacists who are in perfectly happy relationships with fellow Pharmacists attack me venomously, please, this is a little fun. I am aware of very happy partnerships, have even attended weddings of such successful partnerships, but it did get me thinking about the following. I thought about all the strange things Pharmacists ask each other. It's like talking about the weather with everyone else. We seem to have a standard set of questions we ask each other and I just wondered why.

The following is to be read with a pinch of salt, a packet of sarcasm and a hint of irony.

Once a month, Friday night is speed dating night in the LPC venue. There gathers a group of highly attractive, intelligent, single Pharmacists, each hopeful that they'd meet their Mr or Mrs Right that evening. They'd been on other dates, but failed to find anyone who shared their keen passion for Pharmacy. Each had 3 minutes to ask the most important questions they could in order to glean if they were the one for them. Here are those questions:

1] Which university did you go to? – better ask this first in case a) I know them and can't remember them b) I now remember you and my mate dated you in the first year c) the university is important, what if they went to one of those lower, less austere Schools of Pharmacy – the humiliation. We could never make that work.

2] When did you qualify? - It is a question that Pharmacists ask. Why is this? Does this tell us how clever they are? How respected they are? How much money they earn? – We ask it all the same.

I think people often hide behind this. You can meet the 'Newly Qualified/Junior Pharmacist" who uses being new as an excuse for their naivety or their reluctance to make ethical decisions. They ask silly questions and include where they work in their Twitter bio and slate their company/colleagues/managers.

Or you get the "I've been qualified for 28 years". These can seem safe and yet are so deadly. That often translates to "I am an old cynic who qualified 28 years ago, but I've moaned constantly about Pharmacy 'not being like it used to be' for the last 15 years." Be warned, this type can resemble The Death Eaters in Harry Potter. The suck every ounce of passion and enthusiasm you had for Pharmacy out of you in a matter of minutes.

Either way, it's best to ask this question and if necessary, have prepared some additional probing questions to check whether you should duck out here and now from what remains of your 3 minutes.

3] Where do you work? – Here is the contentious one. Do they work in community and thus have no clinical knowledge, not like a hospital Pharmacist? Could I be in a relationship with them? Or maybe they're a Hospital Pharmacist? They have specialist clinical knowledge (in their field), but none of them ever have to make ethical decisions like Community Pharmacists do. The doctors in the hospitals always are there to lend a hand. How would that influence our parenting skills?

Or imagine. What if they work for a large multiple – the shame? Or worse still, they could be a locum – how would I live that down?

4] How busy is your Pharmacy, how many 'items' do you do? – Why do community Pharmacists insist on discussing items like it's some sort of Olympic achievement.

"We do 8000 items a month and I'm the only Pharmacist"

"Well, once I did 400 in a day with one dispenser off sick."

"That's nothing; I once did 400 in a day with a dispenser off sick, my broken leg and an eye patch on"

Surely though if I ask this question I'll know if they're made of stronger stuff?

5] Do you have a Clinical Diploma? – Again, what a bizarre question, but we find ourselves asking it. I wondered if people ask it because they believe those Pharmacists who have Clinical Diplomas are 'proper' Pharmacists. It's obviously best to check because then, if they say yes, you'll know they are a dedicated Pharmacist. If they say no, you can confidently exclude them from your list of hopefuls.

6] Last but not least......Do you know Mr Dispenser? This is a new addition to any Pharmacy conversation I have had of late. The fascination with this person is the new Pharmacy must ask question. And if you say "Yes, I do", well there is a fair chance you'll get a tick and the chance of a proper date. Everyone wants to meet someone who knows Mr Dispenser....don't they?

So, your 3 minutes is up. You've asked those all important questions and it's time to decide. Will there be a second 'date' or is it 'cheerio'?? The decision is yours!

Perils of the Language Barrier by Merlvin Moyo

We've all been in this awkward situation. Standing in front of you is a patient from a foreign country. You speak one language (English in this case); and they speak another. They can't speak one word of your language and as for you, well, you can't even tell where they've come from. If you're in luck, they've brought along a friend or family member that has a rudimentary command of your language.

And so the "consultation" begins, first between the healthcare assistant (HCA) and the patient's rep:

HCA: *'Hi there. Can I help you?'*

Rep: *'Good afternoon. We see pharmacist.'*

HCA: *'Yes ... That is the pharmacist. ... Oh! I'm sorry. Do you want to see the pharmacist?'*

Rep: *'Yes! Yes!'*

HCA: *'Please hold on. I'll get him for you.'*

And so you put on your most helpful face, having heard most of the preceding conversation between the HCA and the patient's rep.

Pharmacist: Good afternoon. I'm John the pharmacist. How can I help you?

Rep (to patient in unknown language): !&2$* %43£@~#

Patient nods and looks at you, then opens mouth and speaks several words in rapid succession,

"!"£$&^*)(@##<! ¬`'¬~~" <?"£%^."

You return a puzzled expression and shake your head from side to side to indicate that you don't understand. You hope that this is not confused with understanding as you are aware that in some cultures the nod and the shaking of the head from side to side have opposite meanings to those in yours. You find yourself turning to the rep and saying slowly and deliberately,

"I. Don't. Understand."

"Ah!" responds the rep, before turning to the patient and explaining the predicament.

The patient begins to gesticulate, rubbing the abdomen between the midriff and pelvic area as well as the derrière.

"Belly. Behind. Painful." adds the rep helpfully.

"Great!" you find yourself thinking. "Now we've narrowed it down to constipation, heartburn, piles, cystitis or any of a number of other possibilities. Am I expected to take my pick and hope for the best?"

You realise that this would not be good patient care. You are also aware of the challenge you face getting a reasonably complete patient history: What medical conditions does the patient suffer from? What is the history of the present condition? What have they already tried for it? What other medication are they taking? Do they have any allergies? Are these new or old symptoms? Have they ever been treated for this before?

You realise you need help. Having someone who can translate more effectively than the rep would be very helpful at this stage. In desperation, you ask the question,

"Do you have any form of identification?"

Both the rep and the patient return blank expressions.

"I'm sorry. Do you have passports?"

"Ah! Passports!" and the documents are immediately fished out of one of the bags that either the patient or the rep is carrying. If not the passport, then a Home Office ID Card is usually provided.

It is at this point that you silently breathe a sigh of relief as you know you can call the PCT and get help through being directed to the language interpretation/translation services.

But wait, this is after the 1st of April 2013! Who can I call for help?

Somebody?

Anybody?

Help!

HELP!

12 Days of Pharmacy

By Molly-Anne Perfect, Kay Perfect, Sachin Kapila, Jamie Carter and Chris Smith

On the 12th day of Christmas my colleagues moaned to me...

12 minutes till closing

11 addicts twitching

10 GP's bleating

9 Loonies laughing

8 Dispensers dispensing

7 tablets missing

6 computers crashing

5 EHC's

4 Children crying

3 Prescriptions not ready

2 Urgent deliveries

and a Zomorph discrepancy

Irish Village Pharmacy by Dr Sheetal Billy Marwaha

In the not too distant past I had the good fortune to secure a summer Locum placement in a border town in Ireland, Unbeknown to myself this town or should I say, Irish Village, was home to several fervent Irish Republicans. It was pointed out to me by one of my golfing partner friends that I ought to visit the place, under his guidance first. When asked why, I was advised that I would probably be the first and last Scouse speaking Asian to appear in the town. Thinking that this had a ring of truth to it, I proceeded to ring the pharmacy to speak to the family of pharmacists that owned the pharmacy.

I was greeted with glee and joy by the retired father, who then told me that I came with lots of references? I was not aware that it was customary to ask other folk about my credentials. He then told me I had the nickname of King Billy from Liverpool and wore a turban! Nevertheless, he was not going to put that against me and that I ought to visit the pharmacy.

The following day armed with my map and compass I made it through the mountainous terrain to the village pharmacy. In short, I was shown around the village shops and their owners and several of the village people, I was then given a lunch allowance to eat anywhere in the village. If I did not have enough money to eat I was told to say I was the Chemist working at Maguire's Pharmacy and I would be seen to free of charge. Only one provision was that I was not allowed to drink more than 3 pints of Guinness at lunchtime.

Midway with my new locum vacation whilst working in the pharmacy, I heard a knock on the back door of the pharmacy. On-going to the door and opening it, I saw a calf roped up to the pharmacy drain pipe. Thinking nothing of it I closed it. Going back to work, I was confronted by a rather rustic looking farmer with an incomprehensible Irish rural accent. The staff then proceeded to translate for me, apparently it was Gaelic he was speaking and no wonder I couldn't understand the vernacular. He wondered if the "man from the big city" could see to his sick calf. Now realising the connection between the knock on the door and the farmer, the man came round the counter to show me his sick animal. The calf had a cough and was keeping the family awake since it slept in the living room.

The BNF had no doses or meds for animals and I was torn between giving a gallon of simple linctus or pholcodine syrup. I thought better and swallowed my pride to ask the retired owner who lived upstairs. The owner then pulled out a wee brown bottle from a disused washing machine and handed it to me and told me to tell the man, one dose today and one dose tomorrow. I then passed on the message to the farmer who happily walked on his merry way.

The following day the same knock on the door happened and this time I saw two brown chickens tied up to the drain. I instantly recognised this as this being for the retired owner,, On calling the owner, who rushed to the door and said that he was expecting a sheep for dinner but chickens will do. This was payment for treating the sick calf!

Over my dead body by Mark Robinson

This blog is written on the day that NICE publishes their Best Practice Guide. With sadness it may mean the end of 'over my dead body' formulary rejection letters - a source of great fun or embarrassment depending on your point of view. I should really write a book, but will it ever be as funny as Mr Dispenser? - I doubt it.

Today, I had a real doozy. An application for Circadin and here are the reasons for rejection:

'Unlicensed indication in over 75' - actually license says over 55 - just let me check - yes 75 is over 55.

'It is unlicensed in hospital inpatients' – hmmm, is there any medicine licensed specifically in inpatients? - do they expect medicines not to work in hospital. Lost for words!

'Difficult to determine a tight cohort' - after all primary insomnia is difficult to diagnose, particularly if you are a Consultant Physician Care of the Elderly - never seen it before - probably needs to be a real expert.

'It would be challenging to not prescribe on discharge' - yes - consultants won't understand - give 7 tablets on discharge and ask the GP to review, stop and give something else.

'Not recommended for GPs to continue' - what does this mean? GPs obviously aren't experienced in insomnia and aren't capable of prescribing one tablet an hour before bedtime for up to 13 weeks. Might as well insult the GPs at the same time!

But after the 'over my dead body' a glimmer of hope...'you can always approach the manufacturer and ask them to sponsor a small in-house trial'. I did say a glimmer of hope - oh no it's gone. Bugger off the answer's no.

Oh well I guess that the only option is to give some temazepam - oh no that's another 'over my dead body' medicines, but at least there is some logic to that one.

If you find another 'over my dead body' rejection, please send it to me - I have a nice collection now.

SOCIAL MEDIA 3

How much?

I feel like a magician sometimes. I can turn 3000ml of Gaviscon Advance into 300ml after a 10second chat with a GP and the magic words, 'Um, can you have a look at this quantity please?' What's the most inappropriate quantity of a medicine that you have seen prescribed (accidentally)?

@MrDispenser A GP once told me that he wasn't a mathematician when I queried a quantity.

1] Jenna R: 28ml of ensure plus milkshake style!

2] Kylie M: 12000 methadone tablets!

3] Liz H: And just this last week, 1000ml of calpol, when I rang the GP to query amount he said *"It's to share between all the children."*

4] Gilli M: 1ml of ensure but the doctor wanted mixed flavours.

5] Jenny E: 21 Microgynon ED, last week. Surgery couldn't work out why that wasn't right.

6] Jo B: 1ml Doublebase

7] Louise T: 1015 diazepam 2mg!!

8] Francesca B: 10 Levonelle

9] Viren S: I had 425 loaves of bread.

10] Zahara A: Naproxen 500mg tablets 28000000 for my dad

11] Martina S: 1000 mL Locorten Vioform

12] Zainab N: 56 Symbicort inhalers on a batch with six repeats!

13] Mark A: 200 Clenil inhalers.

14] Lindsay W: 228 zopiclone tablets

15] Wesley L: 500 codeine tabs

16] Stevie H: 3 Cerazette

17] Nilima P: 566 omeprazole 20mg caps

18] Isla D: Nasonex send (140)

19] Gabriel B: Tobramycin 620kg, iv

20] Lynn S: 20ml lactulose, six 5ml spoonful's nocte for two weeks.

A-Z of Drug Names

Thanks to Stewart Kelly

A

Aimee M: **AIMEE**odarone

Stefi H: **ANNA**strozole

B

Gemma G: **BEN**droflumethiazide

Babir M: pheno**BABIR**tol

C

@littlechloe15: **CHLOE**amphenicol

Joy D: Co-**CAROL**dopa

D

Dawn R: **DAWN**epezil

Joy D: **DIANA**zepam

E

ELLEste Solo

F

FINNasteride

G

Stewart K: **GABI**pentin

Stewart K: **GEMMA**fibrozil

H

@motali86: **HARRY**piprazole

I

Ian S: flucloxasilly**IAN**

@richardbogle: **IVOR**bradine

J

Josephine L: Ben**JO**flumethiazide

Jayne M: **JANE**uvia

K

Katie H: **KATE**oprofen

Katie D: **KATIE**mine

L

Laura M: **LAURA**zepam

Sharon S: **LANCE**zoprazole

M

Lynsey C: **MIKE**ophenolate

@Glamoureyesme: Fosa**MAX**

N

Khalil A: **NICOLA**randil

O

Stefi H: Fur**OZZY**mide

P

Pradeep G: Phenoxymethyl **PENNY**cillin

Q

@MrDispenser: **QUINN**alapril

R

Rani R: **RANI**tidine

Rabia K: **RABIA**prazole

S

Sally W: **SALLY**cylic acid

Sarah L: **SARAH**tide

T

Tamlyn W: **TAMI**flu!

Joy D: Fluoxe**TINA**

U

@MrDispenser: Acenoco**UMA**rol

V

@MrDispenser: **VERA**pamil

Robert B: Sodium **VAL**proate

X

@MrDispenser: E**XENA**tide

Y

Si B: Ami**YODA**rone

Jonny K: **YASMIN**

Z

Zöe H: **ZOE**piclone

Patent Expiry

Mr Dispenser's Blog™ brand of statin is about to lose its patent in a couple of weeks. This is a blockbuster drug for us. As a result, our R + D department are proud to launch some exciting new products:

Blog Fastmelts™

Blog XL™

Blog Mesilate™

Blog Sachets™

Blog Suppository™

Blog Pessary™

Blog injection™

Blog Inhaler™

Thanks to **@andychristo** and **@RSDave** for their ideas

Dispensing

Awkward moment when the dispenser is getting some medicines from the top shelf beside you and you fear for your life and a tablet avalanche.

Ancient Chinese proverb: one who can catch falling prescription before it hits the floor can achieve anything.

You know that a box of tablets has been on the shelf for a while when it has turned a different shade/colour.

It's good that you stick labels on tubes and not on the box but why put the tube back in the box and then give it to me to check?

I always seem to leave the tab out on my own meds once I start a box at home.

Accidentally endorsed a prescription twice and got blurred vision.

There are some really messed up people in this world. Why would you stick on a label upside down? UPSIDE DOWN! WHY WOULD YOU DO THAT? WHY?

Seen those 'Your Speed' signs that tell you how fast you are driving? Installing one at work so staff can see how slow they work.

Awkward moment when you try and help dispense and see a prescription for 84 Stugeron and casually move on to the next prescription.

Steve T: "Getting generics in super-size packaging when the space on the shelves won't accommodate them... Argh!!!"

Brendan K: When I was a young lad, I used to help out as a dispenser in my brother-in-law's pharmacy in Leeds. We had very high shelves. We had a lady locum pharmacist. She insisted on getting some meds from the highest shelf, using these wobbly stepladders. I heard the sound of shelves collapsing, just in time to catch the pharmacist before she hit the floor. However, being human, I couldn't catch the 1000 bright yellow bisacodyl tablets skittering off in all directions.

@aptaim: Anyone else in pharmacy love getting the 500g bottle of Doublebase gel out and making it wobble a bit?

@dodgychemist: Dear Dispensers, Don't walk off like you've done me a favour after putting one box of Amlodipine in a basket. It's not going to label itself.

@stephysilk: Splitting another pack when there's plenty in one already split does my head in!! It's so annoying

@selinahuihoong: I am always the one fetching from the tallest shelf because I am the tallest

@REENABARAI: Don't you just love it when you pour out exactly the right number of tabs onto the counting triangle! It's like a pharmacy hole in one!

Medicines

@MrDispenser: I have seen this on Twitter and apologise as I can't remember where: "Escitalopram is the Mexican version of citalopram."

@MrDispenser: Do we need to fill out a Yellow card for the people who say that they rattle due to number of meds?

@MrDispenser: Never has a product summed up certain people more so than 'Thick and Easy powder.'

@MrDispenser: Life would be simpler if the naming of drugs followed how hurricanes are named. Although Dick would be exempted. "I've ran out". "Not had any today..." "I can't swallow."

@MrDispenser: Adcal-D3 and Irn Bru does not equal Adcal D3 Dissolve.

@MrDispenser: If you get a patient who sounds like he could get abusive because the surgery didn't issue his Viagra this month, then saying 'Come and have a go if you're hard enough' may not be appropriate.

@PatelSuk: Look of horror on women's face when they pick up 1st Rx for a IUD with the huge packaging!

David Shalcross: A lady who wanted a particular brand of flucloxacillin capsules. Apparently this brand worked well last time and as she'd found differences between brands of other medication she wanted the same again. She only had the blister strip that didn't have the brand name on so we ordered one of each from AAH of what they had. None resembled the one she had. She revealed that she is a diviner and would decide which ones to get by divining. She went for a colourful pack of TEVA ones eventually.

@MrDispenser: When life gives you lemons, squeeze some onto Adcal-D3 Tutti Fruiti

@shippingorder: We've got a ghost box of contraceptive tablets that haunts our dispensary. We've come to call it the Marie Cilest.

@MrDispenser: I can mix liquid antibiotics no problem but struggle with hot chocolate.

@MrDispenser: I cry when I get a prescription for 56 MST tablets. Please be kind GPs. 4 more tablets won't kill them (hopefully).

@MrDispenser: Awkward moment when you give out your home number instead of work number and Mrs Dispenser has to explain why we want our quota of Cialis increasing.

@MrDispenser: If I have a decision to make at work, I play Sudocrem tub, repeat-slip, scissors.

@MrDispenser: Do people on Temazepam count how many sleeps there are until their next prescription?

@Basienools: A woman wanted to swap her Nitromin for a Nitrolingual as it fitted in her handbag better.

@CrazyRxMan: With all the Cialis and Viagra I dispensed this New Year weekend, you'd think men only get action once a year!

@SowTomorrow: Customer : *"I'm not taking those tablets, I Googled them, it said they had a long half-life, that doesn't mean they're radioactive does it?"*

@Melchem118: Just been given a secret recipe to make the perfect fish bait. And the secret ingredient is Codeine Linctus. Great excuse.

@AmandaHepburn88: Just got asked if we make the gluten free bread in the back shop!

@jaiminthakrar: I made a patient cry because I refused to supply her with diazepam without a prescription. She then called me "institutionalised". I'd been qualified less than a week...

@MrDodgyChemist: Don't you hate it when you pre-pay for loads of Isosorbide Mono. 10mg/20mg from a new Nigerian supplier who emailed you and it never arrives?

@MrDodgyChemist: Trazodone out of stock! Watch nursing home residents fight back as they finally awake from their slumber and overthrow evil regimes.

@MrDodgyChemist: Instructions to mix up Erythroped PI suspension said to 'Agitate dry granules'. So I told them Simvastatin thinks it's really nosy and annoying.

@MrDodgyChemist: The lump in your throat that forms and the more happier life seems to become, when you get an Rx for Trimethoprim and quantity says FOURTEEN.

@MrDodgychemist: *'Why is my prescription for Temazepam not ready!?' 'We called it out, there was no reply.' 'Oh sorry, I must have fallen asleep.'*

@MrDodgyChemist: *'Pick a number between three and seven inclusive.' 'Five.' 'Your course of Trimethoprim will be five days! Next please.'*

OTC

@MrDispenser: If I ask you a question and you reply by saying, *"Its ok, I have medical training"* that means you went on a first aid course once and failed.

@MrDispenser: Once bitten, twice a day hydrocortisone cream.

@MrDispenser: Getting in the way of a co-codamal addict and his Solpadeine Plus is slightly less scary than getting in the way of a dispenser and her biscuits.

@MrDispenser: Anybody else play 'The OTC product that we will be recommending this week is the one with the shortest expiry date' game?

@MrDispenser: I hope we never sell generic Frontline. I can't be doing with fussy dogs who only want the good stuff, giving me dirty looks.

@checkedshoes: Dear world, if I could sell you a cure for the common cold I would not be working on a Sunday.

@MrDispenser: When I am in the mood to treat myself, I buy Calpol 6+ suspension, instead of paracetamol tabs for my headache.

Jade T: Patient: *"Can I have two boxes of co-codamol please?"* (32s).

Me: *"I'm afraid, one is the legal limit."*

Patient: *"Does this help?"*

He pulls out a card to show he's a chiropodist!

Me: *"I'm afraid not!"*

@MrDispenser: Good cop/bad cop isn't an appropriate OTC questioning technique.

Kevin M: I once misheard a customer who I thought had asked for Ovex, but had actually asked for Otex. The peculiar look I got when I suggested that all members of the household should use the medicine at the same time gave it away!

Michelle D: I was a 17 year old student working in a community pharmacy when a young couple came in and asked for something for 'the morning after'. I went bright red and mumbled that they would need to speak to the pharmacist. I told the pharmacist that the couple had come in for the morning after pill so off he went with his list of sexual health questions. Was pretty embarrassing for the couple, the pharmacist and in particular ME when they clarified they just wanted something for a hangover!

Jess H: I sold a man some Tyrozets once and he asked if they would only numb his throat or his whole body.

Counter Resistance: A man who came in looking for "a tube of something". It quickly became apparent that he had no ideas what he was looking for and he circumnavigated all questions about his symptoms. The pharmacist tried in vain to understand what he needed but the man was stubbornly guessing names of made-up creams and ointments. It eventually boiled down to him saying *"Name some creams and I'll tell you if that's the one,"* The pharmacist and I looked at one another before saying *"No."*

@katjack7: Patient: *"My children have nits".*

Me: *"How old are they?"*

Patient: *"The nits, I don't know?"*

Me: *"No sir, the children".*

@sivani_: Prolonging the WWHAM questions when someone is wearing nice aftershave/perfume. I have issues.

@Xrayser: Man just came in and said *"We need some nit treatment."*

Jane*: "How many are you treating?"*

Man*: "Don't know - they're a bit small to count."*

@LinziBrianMusic: A customer asked me for a non-drowsy sleeping tablet last week.

@MrDodgyChemist: Lady buys Alli regularly for weight loss.

'You've lost weight' I said as she bought another box.

'Really?'

'Yeah your wallet's £60 lighter.'

@MrDodgyChemist: What did the codeine addict say to the pharmacist? Don't be silly, they never need to go past the healthcare assistant.

@MrDodgyChemist: Sold some Nytol last week. Guy came in today. I asked how he found it. He said he slept like a baby. He soiled himself twice, woke up crying.

Katharine C: We have a man that comes in to buy Paramol repeatedly and then when we say no he says it's because he has a metal plate fitted and he's in pain. However, depending on which member of staff serves him, the plate moves position... hand, foot, head, arm, leg.

SERVICES

MURs

@MrDispenser: I wanted to do an MUR on an 84 year old lady. She met all the criteria and was waiting but I did not know if it was her that was waiting or a rep. Staff were not sure either. She had not ticked the appropriate box on her prescription. She kind of looked 84 but could have been in her late 60s. Once people reach a certain age, it's hard to guess their age.

@JemimaMcC: Don't you just hate being c.c into an email from the regional manager thanking your line manager for MURs like it's them who do them!

@MrDodgyChemist: Just done a high risk MUR on a claustrophobic serial killer.

@MrDispenser: Awkward moment when you have to sneakily text a pre-agreed code word to your tech to come and get you when a patient won't stop talking during a MUR.

@MrDodgyChemist: *'Would you be interested in making the pharmacy £28 Mr Allen?' 'What do I have to do?'*

'Nothing. Just sign here.'

@MrDispenser: Targeted MUR on Diclofenac. Don't judge me. They all count. Don't hate the playa, hate the game.

@MrDodgyChemist: Doing MUR and drug popped up that I've never heard of. Used the old *'And do you know what this is for?'* chestnut. Patient was blank. Useless!

@MrDispenser: Just saw one of my patients at the supermarket and had a sneaky look at her shopping trolley. I made a mental note to discuss level of chocolate biscuit consumption at next MUR.

@MrDispenser: I got asked during an MUR if we get paid extra for doing them. I gave a politician's answer!

@MrDodgyChemist: *'Can I have a quick word about your medication?*

'I'm busy right now I'll do it next time'

'OK, we still owe you a box so how about tomorrow?'

@MrDispenser: It's not the size of your yearly MUR total that counts; it's how you use them.

@MrDodgyChemist: *'You told me it would be here by this afternoon!' 'Yes you're right but didn't I also tell you to lose some weight during an MUR last year?'*

@MrDispenser: Big spider spotted in consultation room. MURs suspended until further notice.

@MrDodgyChemist: The best thing about having celebrity patients is that you can get their autograph and do an MUR with just one swish of their pen.

@MrDispenser: Two MURs a day, keeps the Area Manager away.

@MrDispenser: How do you make a 95 year old laugh? Give them healthy lifestyle advice during an MUR.

@MrDispenser: That awkward moment your MUR takes longer than expected and staff start wondering if there is a hostage situation.

@MrDispenser: I had my technician bullying me NOT to do any more MURS that day as it was the end of the month and she had already filled out the FP34C.

@sivani_: Did an MUR with a lady in her 90's today. She ended up giving me advice!

@MrDispenser: Awkward moment when you realise that staff have been searching for 10+ item MURs for you to do, just so you get out of their way for a bit!

@MrDispenser: Just asked an old man if he gets any bruising with his warfarin. He said *'only when the wife starts on me'*

@MrDispenser: When discussing grapefruit juice interactions, don't forget to mention Lilt.

@Fosserider: Working in a branch that has done 400 MURs by mid-March already is effing brilliant! Two weeks grace

@MrDispenser: My locum did 10 MURs today which proves that I should sit at home in my pyjamas on Twitter all day more often.

@MrDodgyChemist: How do you confuse a pharmacist? Tell him/her there's a patient who wants to have an MUR and watch as he/she struggles to compute the information.

@MrDispenser: If patients are staying away from the pharmacy due to rain then surely the MUR yearly target should be recalculated using Duckworth-Lewis?

@MrDodgyChemist: *'Can I have a quick chat with you about your meds?'*

'No.'

'Can you just sign here so we don't ask you again for another year?'

Keep it Simple Stupid

Sometimes, the more you explain something, the less enticing it becomes.

Me: *"Hi, Mr Smith. Can I do a MUR on you please?"*

Mr Smith: *"You what?"*

Me: *"Medicines use review"*

Mr Smith: *"What the hell are you on about, boy?!?"*

Me: *"Just want a quick chat about your medicines."*

Mr Smith: *"Why, what's wrong?"*

Me: *"Nothing hopefully"*

Mr Smith: *"I speak to my GP about my medicines"*

Me: *"Yes, I know. I would like to speak to you too about them."*

Mr Smith: *"Are you saying I can't trust him?"*

Me: *"Noooo! I just want to see how you are doing with them."*

Mr Smith: *"Doing fine"*

Me: *"I want to see if you know what they are all for"*

Mr Smith: *"You calling me stupid?!?"*

Me: *"Um…ah.. No. It's just a quick check to see if you are taking them as prescribed"*

Mr Smith: *"I am"*

Me: *"It really will just take a few minutes"*

Mr Smith*: "I'm parked in the disabled spot so have no time. Bye."*

How to hit 400 MURs

This is guidance from one of the multiples on how to achieve that 400 target:

1] Patients on none or more tablets are eligible.

2] Don't waste time on the 10 item plus ones. Time is money!

3] When taking a prescription off a patient, ask them if they are alright. If they say yes, BOOM! Put it through as an MUR.

4] No time to do them? Let your summer student have a go.

5] MURs on antibiotics are allowed.

6] Do one on your spouse, children, parents, uncles and Great Aunt Mildred who is 98 and only takes Zopiclone.

7] Babies who use Ibuprofen suspension. Targeted MUR…

8] Ask patient if they want a beer in the consultation room. Once they are trapped, lecture them about drinking.

9] Ask patients if they want some sweets in the consultation room. Once trapped, lecture them about not accepting sweets from strangers.

Interesting MURS

1] Stuart H: *"Do I need to put the inhaler in my mouth when I use it? Or can I just spray it near my face?"* Yes, she was actually using it like perfume.

2] Nicki D: *"I only take my aspirin (75mg) if my legs feel a bit achey and only use my Spiriva inhaler if I'm going out!"*

3] Katy H: *"I don't take my Bendroflumethiazide because it makes me go to the toilet!"*

4] Stacey T: *"I take my warfarin whenever my blood feels thick"*

5] @sarayummymummy: Been asked on numerous occasions for my number, a date etc etc etc!

6] @Beebs_A: Advised a patient about having an active lifestyle, his *response "it's too cold to go out for a walk, would my GP write a script for a treadmill"*

7] @*sue_warman*: Patient told me how much a Devon and Cornwall railcard could save me in a year.

8] @AlmasRay: I was asked how many bowls of Rice Krispies she would need to eat to get her RDI of iron...And it was a serious question!

9] @shalpatz: Wasn't me but a pharmacist spoke to a patient who was adamant that his high cholesterol was due to eating a Gregg's pasty! He then proceeded to rant about how Gregg's should have a public health warning that they cause high cholesterol!

10] @LSD_Locum: A diabetic who wasn't taking his medication told me Jesus was cool with it, so was his GP; didn't understand why I wasn't. Best of it was the GP told the patient the MUR was a waste of money...whilst issuing a prescription for medicines he wasn't taking?

Other Services

Cameron K: This story was told to me by an old pharmacy inspector. In a pharmacy that did onsite pregnancy testing the following occurred. Family bring in a prescription for Calpol or some such for little Johnny on a Friday afternoon. Then get the medicine and go home etc. After the weekend the father comes back and complains that the medicine tastes awful and that little Johnny won't take it under no circumstances, even when all the family take some too to try and persuade him to take it.

Turns out they'd been given somebody's urine sample brought in for a pregnancy test by mistake complete with label for the Calpol or whatever it was. The thought of the whole family drinking someone's urine sample still cracks me up.

Smoking and Lipotrim

@MrDispenser: Annoying moment when you see one of your smoking cessation clients the next day walking past the pharmacy smoking.

@timhames: We've had them drop their cigarette in street and turn and walk other way when they know they've been clocked!

Clare05: Or your Lipotrim diet patient with a pasty from Greggs in their hand.

@MrDispenser: That awkward moment when you've had chips and cheese for your lunch in the consultation room and a Lipotrim patient walks in to be weighed!

EHC

@S9njay: A patient once came in on a Saturday and asked for Levonelle. I asked if she had UPSI in the last 72hours, yes she replies, '5mins ago'!

@MrDispenser: When the GP receptionist rings up to ask if you do the 'morning after pill' for free, absolutely positively do not reply with "Have a good night Barbara, eh?"

@chirpychickk: You should never ask a lady her age unless she comes in for EHC.

@Xrayser: Lots of EHC this morning. "In spring, a young man's fancy turns to love" said Tennyson. Pity it doesn't also turn to contraception.

Minor Ailments

@MrDispenser: My handwriting is terrible. For the record, I supplied Hedrin and not heroin on the minor ailment scheme.

STUDENTS

Pharmacy Exams

Exams for pharmacy students are a time of great stress. However, for the exam invigilators, they are a time of great amusement.

In order to get through the long exam, invigilators take it in turns to stand next to the:

1) Ugliest

2) Best looking

3) Most likely to fail

4) Most likely to be the first to get struck off

5) Most annoying

6) Cleverest

7) Most likely to cry

8) Students that look like lecturers

9) Coolest

10) Student that probably started revising last night

11) Most likely to start a Facebook campaign demanding the resit be easier

12) Most likely to appear on Jeremy Kyle

13) Most likely be the first to complain on Twitter later

14) Most likely to be a homeopath

15) Most likely to study medicine straight after

So be worried if an invigilator stands beside you!

Alternative Oaths

Huddersfield University make their students pledge a pharmacy oath. Here are some alternative pharmacy oaths:

1] @MrDispenser: This pharmacy does not deal with terrorists or people who demand specific generic medicines.

2] @grahamjudas: Thou shalt stop saying 'it does exactly what it says on the tin' every time you see the Anoheal cream.

3] @MrDispenser: Thou shalt not laugh at people who mispronounce drugs.

4] @andychristo: Thou shalt rejoice when the phrase 'Can you hurry it up, I've a taxi waiting' is uttered.

5] @MrDispenser: Thou shall not urinate in the lactulose.

6] @grahamjudas: Thou shalt not laugh at patients with weird names.

7] @MrDispenser: Thou shalt not say *'Google it'* when a patient asks a question.

8] @rikash_p: If you see a customer outside of work avoid eye contact and pretend you did not see them

9] @MrDispenser: Thou shalt not interrupt the counter assistant on a Monday morning when she regales her tales of the weekend.

10] @DonnaMcCormack1: Thou shalt not repeatedly put that patient who always complains' script to the bottom of the pile.

11] @MrDispenser: Thou shalt not say *"And you just killed someone"* when a dispenser gives you 31 paracetamol instead of 32.

12] @DonnaMcCormack1: Thou shalt not kill and stuff a pharmacist and keep him in the dispensary to get 'round the Responsible Pharmacist rules.

13] @MrDispenser: Thou shalt not make fun of the area manager because he used to work at KFC.

14] @andychristo: Thou shalt understand expensive brands are much superior to cheaper medicines.

15] @MrDispenser: Thou shalt not reply 'no' when someone rings up to ask if you are open.

16] @andychristo: Thou shalt not roll thine eyes when patients mention that they found it on the Internet.

17] @MrDispenser: Thou shalt not tweet about the people you meet or write a book about them.

18] @MikeHewitson1: Thou shalt not supply DIY products when a patient asks for Cuprinol. It would be a stain on the profession.

19] @jasonpeett: We offer a free medication interaction advice service for all recent purchases made in Holland and Barrett.

20] @MikeHewitson1: Thou shalt not scream on a Saturday morning when the only item in a 200 line order that you need is missing.

21] @rob_a_mitchell: When over hearing patients saying a product is cheaper at B@%#s thou shalt not scream "f@%k off to B@%#s then."

22] @MikeHewitson1: Thou shalt smile every time you hear the words 'shipping order', even though you are too young to remember what one is.

23] @rob_a_mitchell: Thou shalt not make up "manufacturing delays" because you forgot to order it.

24] @josh6H: Thou shalt not taste thy methadone.

25] @andychristo: Thou shalt not roll thine eyes at patients who complain they're not overweight it's just their metabolism.

26] **@MrDispenser:** Thou shalt not make the dispensers fat by buying them cream cakes

The Life of a Pharmacy Student by Sophie Khatib

Not surprisingly, my drug of choice as a student is caffeine – and I drink coffee almost continuously throughout the day, well, interspersed with diet coke of course! The majority of my days therefore start with a coffee in hand….nothing to do with a constant hangover of course!

Once fully woken up, well as much as can be expected for a student, I grab my notes, books, laptop, prescription folder, journals and of course my trusty BNF (the one with the cover that most matches my outfit, of course!).

Lectures flit from x-ray diffraction to legal issues, ethical problem solving to dispensing, drug formulation to clinical pharmacy and genetic biomarkers to drug biochemistry. Way too much for my brain to handle – more coffee and plenty of note taking….in that order.

After a full day of lectures, it's time to walk home. Normally in the rain – we are in England after all. My priorities have massively changed in the last couple of years – I would rather keep my folder of work dry than my hair. How did I end up in this position?? University is changing me!

The best bit of being a pharmacy student is the huge subject diversity we experience and the great wealth of knowledge we pick up on the way. Having said that, it's very hard work. VERY hard work. I never expected it to be easy but admittedly, never thought it would be quite so intense. It'll all be worth it when I graduate and buy myself that gorgeous pair of Jimmy Choos!

The bit of my education that I most enjoy (apart from going out!!) is having time to do research in my own time. It's really enjoyable looking into something that you found particularly interesting. It's very rewarding when you realise that you have hit the point where you can print out a journal article on a pharmaceutical subject and actually understand it….well most of it. You can't have it all can you – I'm happy with understanding most of it for the time being. There is only so much that coffee can do – I don't think its good enough to perk my brain up that much. It's a miracle that it manages to do what it does. I'd be stuck without it!

Time to go and put the kettle on again….

Alternative OSCE

1] @MrDispenser: You have to make tea for 5 other staff but only have milk for 4 people.

2] Kelly T: The "it's not for me" co-codamol/Nytol station: one out of the 10 patients will be telling the truth- can you spot the right one?

3] Adam P: Persuading a patient that generic is on a par to brand.

4] Emily B: A station where you do 3 stations

5] Andrew P: Explaining to a patient that the repeat slip lists all of their medication not just what was on their prescription and just because something's on the list doesn't mean it was on the prescription.

6] Gina E: Dealing with receptionist station to get to the GP and discuss a clinical query with someone who knows the answer.

7] Stacey T: Being able to know why the person sitting in the waiting area is there, without asking, even though they haven`t come to the counter.

8] Alma A: Justify why the prescription will take 5 minutes - after all, it's just picking up a box off the shelf.

9] Andrew P: Checking a blister pack containing 34 different white round tablets with no markings.

10] Aíslinn M: Measuring for hosiery and trusses.

11] Deborah M: Meeting MUR targets.

12] Aisha A: How to identify the drug by colour they're telling you.

13] Yvonne S: How to identify which patient you are talking to when you answer the phone and they just shout at you to ask if their prescription is ready.

14] Catherine H: Identify the cause of the rash...over the phone.

15] Nasaar A: Manufacturer Cannot Supply station.

16] Kelly T: Lunch speed eating.

17] Jo B: The 'I can't order your medication if you don't know which ones you want' station.

18] Michael M: A station where you have to use your magic wand to produce the obtainable out of thin air. I have been known to use the phrase to a patient *"If I had a magic wand I would wave it"* as recent as yesterday.

19] @phig75: Refilling the ink on the stamp without making a complete mess is difficult.

20] @vari_d: How to get past the surgery receptionists and speak to a doctor.

21] @a_lethal_dose: Fill your mind with enough celeb gossip/X-factor/Eastenders to have a half decent conversation with your dispensary team.

22] @a_lethal_dose: Spend the least amount of time repeating *'the doctor's surgery didn't authorise your repeat'* before the patient gets the hint.

23] @svwild: The 'Codeine addict' or 'the patient that knows exactly what's wrong with them from Google' station.

24] @StephenLunn1: Knowing what size truss to order by sight?

25] @StephenLunn1: Ability to remember and make the tea/coffee preferences of a dozen staff members.

Look it up

@MrDispenser: Awkward moment when the university student asks me a question I don't know and I tell them to look it up in the BNF.

David M: I tell them to look it up in the Drug Tariff. Keeps them quiet longer, and you can guarantee they'll never ask you an awkward question ever again.

Laura W: Then when they tell you the answer you nod along like you knew the whole time.

Ann P: I just tell 'em I don't know. And to look it up, then tell me the answer. The way I see it is I'm both old and quite clever, so if I've never needed to know then it's probably not that important. Mind you, that's now I'm old and confident. Newly qualified I'd have probably gone with the classic "well I could tell you, but you'll learn so much more from finding it out on your own..." This has the additional benefit of being true, well the second bit, anyway!

Amanda H: When the pharmacist says "look it up" we all know it's because you don't have a clue what the answer is.

Jenny E: It encourages them to undertake self-directed learning. That's what I tell them to cover my ignorance.

Claire W: I like to answer these questions with *"Do I look like the BNF?"* works a treat!

Andy C: That's almost the stock answer to any question asked by a student / pre-reg. *"Where do you think you would find the answer?"*

Students

@Xrayser: What is it about students? Just done CO reading on 3 of them for Stop Smoking Service and the one whose reading is off the scale punches the air in victory

@MrDispenser: Awkward moment when the male summer student makes a sexist joke and tries to high-five me but I have already dived over the counter and assumed the foetal position in fear of my safety.

Hannah: Awkward moment when asked by a fellow student if the oral contraceptive was used for incidences of JUST oral coitus.

@kaymklee: The couple sat directly in front of me need to get a room. I'm trying to study. No public displays of affection in the library, please.

@ronagandhi: Got my first library warning today because I was talking about Bonjela in the silent area.

@5anaan: Note to self: when asked *"What is the role of Pharmacist in hospital?"* Don't say *"holding the BNF"* I had a narrow escape.

@miss_njun: That sudden urge for a celebratory dance when you see that question you were so badly hoping for.

@AmmarahShafia: Steal of the day: 13 pregnancy tests. How many women did you knock up?! He came back 2 hours later and pinched a bunch of baby wipes. Guess the results were positive!

@jaanki_: A man asked for my number whilst buying 24 condoms. I don't know if he's a prick or just really confident?

Maryam A: I got offered an interview for Moorfields Eye hospital summer placement, I was abroad at the time so I wanted email to find out whether or not they could give me a Skype or phone interview, and sorry for any inconvenience. To my despair AFTER I got told no, I realised I had originally typed sorry for any incontinence I may have caused you instead of inconvenience to the head of pharmacy at the hospital.

@noureenfazal: Awkward moment when you realize you have been taking your asthma inhaler wrong all these years.

@bethevans92: I can't even pronounce the names of some drugs, how am I meant to learn all about them.

Al J: "Our university cafe charges 90p for a cup of tea. In second year I discovered a loophole combining the 10p discount for using your own cup and them only charging 20p for a cup of hot water. Initially, people mocked me for carrying tea bags and a thermos to uni every day - now I see loads of people doing it!"

@weeneldo: I could read the BNF, but I already know how it ends (abbreviations and symbols, Latin abbreviations then E numbers).

@MrDodgyChemist: FAO students struggling with calculations - Patient comes with 12 item walk-in. How long does HCA say it will be a) 3 minutes b) 4 minutes or c) NOW?

Andy C: When I was a student we had a pharmacist who used to throw dispensing errors back across the dispensary! He was a bit odd!

@MrDispenser: Summer student called technician a Luddite. Technician got upset. She doesn't know what a Luddite is.

ANNOYED

How to annoy your pharmacist

1] @ApothecaryTales: Tell me it's cheaper at Walmart.

2] @kung_fu_pandya: Buy a 20 pack of cigs and then come to get some paracetamol tabs on the Minor Ailments Scheme for free.

3] @J_AI_S: Ask about animal medicines.

4] @sam4715: It's on the repeat so it must be on the prescription.

5] @theancientartof: Shouting 'OY LADY! You in there! Where's my prescription?'

6] @phuriouspharmer: When you call out "Mary Smith" and a man says "Yes, well not literally" cracks me up.

7] @LSD_Locum: When they hand a prescription with 20 urgent items 2 minutes before closing.

8] @EmmTurner: You: *'Do you take any other medication?'* Patient: *'It's ok- my wife/husband is a nurse.'*

9] @ApothecaryTales: Try to return a used bag of pancake mix you bought up front 4 years ago.

10] @ApothecaryTales: Joking that you just printed it when someone checks to see if your 50's a fake.

11] OneMissSharan: *"Can I speak to your pharmacist dear?"*

12] @shn86: *'The locum we had yesterday was quicker at checking off and he was fitter too.'*

13] @ApothecaryTales: Say *"Wow, it's so nice outside, sucks you have to work."*

14] @Cleverestcookie: *'Can I speak to the pharmacist?'* Looking past you at the older male tech in the background (happened to me).

15] @ApothecaryTales: Say you used to work in a pharmacy.

16] @andychristo: Let your kids run into my dispensary and shout at me when I try and stop them eating the diazepam.

17] @andychristo*: "Do you take any other medicines?"* *"No" "What about the carrier bag you've just picked up?"* *"That doesn't count."*

18] @residentlocum: Ask him if he watched X-Factor/Celebrity Jungle/any other bullshit TV show.

19] @andychristo: *"I've got the flu!"* No you don't! If you had flu, you wouldn't be able to walk into the store and tell me!

20] @andychristo: Patient handing back unused meds *"Do you know how much these cost?" "It's OK son, I don't pay for prescriptions."*

21]@andychristo: *"Are you taking any other medication?" "It's OK, I've had it before."*

22] @andychristo: *"Are you taking any other medication?" "Yes, a white one, two blue ones and another thingy one."*

23] @andychristo: *"Are you taking any other medication?" "None of your business."*

24] @Mexican_Badger: Ask *"Is the usual pharmacist not here?"*

25] @residentlocum: Complain because you have to wait 20 minutes because the pharmacist is on a lunch break. Why do they need to eat anyway?

26] @andychristo: Ask me: *"Did you not get into medical school?"*

27] @shn86: When a patient says very loudly *'I will have you know that I am a Dr, I know what I'm doing.'*

28] @andychristo: Complain to me when I recommend that you need to see your GP.

29] @andychristo: Start shouting at my staff.

30] @andychristo: Come in with a new script for the same drug you handed 20 boxes of back yesterday.

31] @andychristo: *'Are you waiting or calling back for this prescription?' 'Yes.'*

32] @jaysonjaz: Call up and ask for drugs by their street names.

33] @theancientartof: Kick off as prescription not delivered a) we haven't got your prescription b) you've never used our dispensing services before.

34] @theancientartof: *'I've come to pick up my prescription' 'What name is it?' 'Jane'* Of course we always file Rx by first names.

35] @rmoomin1: Hand in a script with unidentifiable stains on it.

36] @MrDispenser: Pay for your prescription using 1p and 2p's.

37] @residentlocum: Don't introduce yourself or ask their name. Just demand MURs and NMS.

38] @MrDispenser: Say, *'I have been waiting 45 mins for the doctors but I refuse to wait 10 minutes for my prescription.'*

39] @MrDispenser: Throw a tube of Smarties at them and say, *'Count this.'*

40] @rmoomin1: *'I've got a taxi waiting outside'* or the hospital version *'There's an ambulance already booked.'*

How to annoy rival 100 hour pharmacy

1] @MrDispenser: Ring them and ask if they have done a prescription for Hugh Jass.

2] @MrDodgyChemist: Tell all the local tramps that there's somewhere warm with chairs where they can spend most of the week.

3] @MrDispenser: Ring every hour to see if they are open.

4] @MrDodgyChemist: Tell them clocks have gone back so they need to open for 101 hours this week.

5] @MrDispenser: Send in your mum with her 15 item script at 10.59pm.

6] @MrDodgyChemist: Phone and ask if they do enough items to cover their electric bills.

7] @MrDispenser: Send your horrible patients to them.

8] @MrDodgyChemist: Stick a "2 hour waiting time" notice in their window.

9] @MrDispenser: Let pharmacy students know on Twitter and FB that if they ever need any help with coursework or any pharmacy questions then to ring the 100 hour pharmacy.

10] @MrDodgyChemist: When I'm bored I sometimes phone the 100 hour pharmacy and get them to order high value goods for me and promise to bring in a prescription.

PEOPLE

Locums

@MrDodgyChemist: The day always goes so quickly when you turn up late to work. As a locum, I'm often late for work. I say often, I mean every day. I got a kick up the arse today though when someone stole my parking spot.

@MrDodgyChemist: The best thing about locuming isn't the flexibility or money. The best thing is being able to wear the same shirt every day. No one will ever know.

@MrDodgyChemist: Which dispensing system do locums most prefer? I like the one where the dispenser dispenses, I check and someone else bags up and gives out.

@MrDispenser: Just popped into one of my old pharmacies for 2 minutes and the locum turned up. I may have pretended for 30secs that we'd been double booked.

@MrDispenser: Locum: Today was so busy I didn't even have time to look at my mobile for an hour!

@MrDispenser: What do you do as manager if you find out that you have had a crap locum and they are related to you? Tell Locum Agency or tell their Dad?

@Shab_Sherni: There's nothing worse than a second cover pharmacist who doesn't talk... I.e. *'so have u travelled far?'* And their response is *"no."*

@Busby_88: At one locum, a little old lady accused me of trying to poison her as I had the gall to give her generic omeprazole.

@impure3: I had a row with a locum over a pill prescription. He was adamant the cc stood for with food

@Checkedshoes: Locum who if the shop was busy would answer the phone with the name of the local police station and then put the phone down.

Rich: There are a couple of locums near me who are identical twins. Very confusing before I realised they were different people

Bianca: I had a guy who would bring in the biggest lunchbox you've ever seen and just eat all day, unplug the fridge to put the radio on, then take his shoes off, sing loud and throw a few shapes in the dispensary when all around him the place was chaos.

Bianca: One locum had the worst toupee you've ever seen. It would gradually move throughout the day.

Andy C: Ever had the newspaper reading locum who got annoyed when asked to check a script?

David F: I worked one day with only one dispenser who refused to talk to me or even acknowledge my existence.

Andy C: I remember one pharmacy I got ignored by the whole staff!

@MrHunnybun: I used to know a locum who took his own kettle and microwave with him. Kept them in his boot and used PRN!

@aptaim: Just had an email-off with another locum who arrived, in a battle to decide who's meant to be working here today. *victorious.*

Staff

@MrDispenser: When on a staff night out, I insist that the staff all wear their work uniform so that if I lose one, they are easy to spot.

@MrDispenser: Awkward moment when you fall asleep whilst waiting for the staff to finish dispensing.

@MrDispenser: Instead of appraisals this year, I will hold a parent's evening and discuss my techs pen stealing with her folks.

@MrDispenser: I said to the tech: *'Your hair looks nice. Have you had a haircut?'*

She said: *'No, just washed it.'*

I said: *'You should do that more often.*

Once I regained consciousness, I took 2 Aspirin for the headache.

@MrDodgyChemist: How to deal with negative staff... ...Bose QC15 noise cancelling headphones.

@MrDispenser: How do you know when it's 5pm in pharmacy? The gush of wind as your tech runs past you to go home for their early finish.

@MrDodgyChemist: How many dispensers does it take to change a light bulb? Just one, providing there is another making the coffee for the mid-task coffee break.

@MrDodgyChemist: Why did the Healthcare Assistant cross the road? She was going home as she only worked 4 hours a day, so her shift was over just as it was getting busy.

@MrDodgyChemist: Following the complaints about hair being found in patients' trays I have made it a rule for everyone to dye their hair different colours.

@MrDodgyChemist: Why did the dispenser cross the road? All the gossip on this side of the road had been exhausted so she was looking for new material.

@MrDispenser: Any day in which I don't have staff on holiday, off sick, suspended, in prison, rehab or witness protection is a good day. I need a full team.

@MrDispenser: You can't beat technicians. I checked in our SOPs.

@MrDispenser: Awesome moment when it's my round to make a cuppa and no one wants one (This is not a reflection on my tea-making. I have had good feedback).

@MrDispenser: I tell my staff to work harder because people on benefits are relying on them.

@MrDispenser: I have three words of advice to dispensers: Please learn to count.

@MrDispenser: Me: *'So how long have you worked here?'* Saturday lad: *'It's my first day'* Me inside: *'Oh crap.'*

@MrDispenser: Awkward moment when you get a script to check and realise that the script is still in the endorser. Do you take the long walk back or send for help?

@MrDispenser: If someone you work with asks *'Why am I here?'*, absolutely positively do not respond with *'Poor life choices.'*

Khalil A: Why is it always that when the staff finish for the day and the remaining dispenser is on lunch...that every Tom, Dick and Harry decide to come into the pharmacy, along with Mr Smith on the phone with a horrible query?..aarghhhh! When the dispenser gets back-it's all died down and they can't see what the fuss was all about!

@MrDispenser: Hell hath no fury like a pharmacy technician scorned.

@MrDispenser: Good to get to know your staff. It helps form a bond. Find out things about them e.g. middle name. Use their full name when they are in trouble.

@MrDodgyChemist: Awkward Moment when you try to join in halfway through a staff conversation and you get a dirty look which says *'do you always listen in?'*

@MrDispenser: 'My doctor says that I should try orlistat but I don't know why' said the dispenser at 9.15 whilst eating her third biscuit and washing it down with Coke.

@MrDodgyChemist: Irony - Two Healthcare Assistants standing around and bitching about how every time they go to Tesco pharmacy, the staff are just standing around talking.

@Genniee_x: Oh I do enjoy spending my lunch hour with patients from work because they've come for a 'natter' at my nans.

@MrDispenser: I used to have a dispenser who didn't dispense until I rang up Trading Standards who came and spoke to them.

@BossARoss: That awkward moment when the tech that we fired yesterday, shows up for his shift today.

@MrDispenser: My staff members are slow at dispensing except when I go to the toilet and come back to 8 prescriptions that need checking.

@Babir1981: One issue with working close to home is the careless redistribution and discussion of information of other people that may or may not be true (aka gossiping). There are no secrets in a community. You need to be careful as anyone could walk through the door while you are in the middle of dissecting Mrs Smith's love life.

@checkedshoes: I only tweet from work for reasons of sanity. I promise not to tweet, if staff do not discuss fake tan, the bits they shave, their sex lives, their children's sex lives, their behaviour when drunk, their husbands behaviour when drunk or shopping.

@MrDispenser: I like to buy edible treats for my staff because they work hard. Another reason is that they may stop talking if their mouth is full.

Kevin M: I counted *21* open pots of Calcichew D3 in one pharmacy I worked in. This is not a joke.

@MrDispenser: Playing 'guess the indication' with staff. It's both enjoyable and depressing with their lack of knowledge. I must stop choosing hard ones.

Rich: No matter how many times you say it: moths are NOT the physical manifestations of spirits. Why do so many dispensers believe in ghosts?

@MrDispenser: 30% of pharmacy staff admit to having problems with their maths when counting tablets. The other 80% said they had no issues.

Alan S: Anne is fond of "finding" and taking an odd diazepam knowing it's a vitamin B tablet. Apparently she once did it with green syrup for methadone. She only owned up to stop the newly qualified pharm from dialling 999.

Kids

@MrDispenser: Awkward moment when you get a prescription for a baby with a unisex name and you don't know which way to label it.

@MrDispenser: Parent of naughty kid in pharmacy pointed today at me and said to son, 'That mister will take you into that small room if you don't behave!' I just stood there trying not to look scary and mentally scarring the kid.

@MrDispenser: *"Just to let you know, this medication may make your child drowsy."*

After hugging me, the parent says *"Thank you!"*

@MrDispenser: How do you shut up a stroppy teenager? Ask them to confirm their address when you hand out their prescription. They always look to their Mum.

@MrDispenser: Amusing when you hand out a prescription for a child and they do not say thanks and the parent tells them off!

@MrDispenser: Awkward moment when Mum comes in for a prescription for two kids for same item and you only have enough for one kid so you ask them who they love the most?

@MrDispenser: I gave a child a MUR sticker today for behaving in the pharmacy. I told him to tell his friends. I'm expecting lots of MUR requests in 10 years. I'm planning for the future.

@MrDispenser: A child today shouted *'Finally!'* upon getting his Amoxicillin suspension. I think he will grow up to be one of those impatient patients.

@MrDispenser: I had a child crying in the pharmacy today and saying *"I don't want to be in the pharmacy, I want to go to bed!!!"* and I nodded in agreement.

@MrDispenser: My new favourite drug side-effect: A 5 year old girl was caught lying by her mum and blamed it on... her asthma inhaler. She is a genius.

@MrDodgyChemist: *'The man said you can't have the lollipop'* said the woman, pointing at me, to her young kid. A complete lie. I would NEVER refuse a sale.

@MrDodgyChemist: Dispensed Metronidazole suspension for a 3 year old and told him to avoid alcohol. Luckily, he had a responsible mum who took his lager away.

@MrDodgyChemist: Dispensed Cetirizine liquid for a 4 year old and told him it may affect his driving reaction time. His mum whipped him off his tricycle.

Elderly

Spencer L: As a newly I once refused sale of Canesten for thrush to a pensioner on a motibility scooter. She asked why and I said because she was over 60. She then came out with the line that will live for me forever *"Young man, would you mind telling me what the difference is between a fanny at 59 and a fanny at 70"?!* I went bright red and replied I had no practical experience.

@lauraberrycakes: I had an elderly lady come in with her hood up due to rain and asked if we allowed hoodies in the shop!

@MrDispenser: There was an old man standing on the counter. I said that I would just be a minute. He said not to rush as the only thing you get from rushing is a baby.

@MrDispenser: Old man asked me if the girls in the pharmacy down the road were better looking. Thought it was better to lie and said *'No'* really loudly.

@MrDispenser: I'm having a sign put up next week: *"During busy periods, only two old people allowed in the pharmacy at any one time."*

@MrDispenser: Awkward moment when the old man realises that his new private prescription for that drug that he wanted is not free.

@MrDispenser: I am going to practice my angry stare for the next twenty years so that I can use it when I am a pensioner in pharmacies.

Kay P: I am going to be that little old lady that has bubbles not blister packs, insist on branded only preferably the pink ones, relate in great detail how things were done in pharmacies in my day, complain that in my day nobody waited more than 5 minutes for their 25 item prescriptions and pretend not to hear my name called so I can sit and have a warm and so save on my heating bills.

@bemyserene_: And when a pharmacist is telling you about your meds you can come out with *"I used to be a pharmacist you know!"*

@OakfieldNo6: I've already planned to be on lots of meds and order one item every three days.

@DotRonnie: Don't forget to include the tutting too!

@jadewatt: And get your speech ready about how you don't want the generic drugs because they are cheap and nasty rip-offs?

SOCIAL MEDIA 4

My Worst Fear

1] @MrDispenser: Running out of tea bags.

2] @MrDispenser: Losing my pen.

3] @MrDispenser: Doctors with good handwriting. It would mean that I would have to stop guessing.

4] @studentpharmacy: Not reading patient titles correctly and getting the sex of the patient wrong!

5] @MikeHewitson1: When you're not sure if a female customer is pregnant, or in need of a public health intervention.

6] @JV_Roberts: Clumsy dispenser spilling Methadone mixture!

7] @cirrusblue2002: Spider in dispensary. Dispensary staff presume incorrectly that token male pharmacist can deal with this.

8] @MrDispenser: The pharmacy robots becoming self-aware and taking over.

9] @MrDispenser: Your former pre-reg opening a pharmacy across the road from you

10] @Pharm_Thoughts: Having 10 people waiting in line with only 2 minutes until closing.

11] @abitina: Finding a script after having a 'barney' with the receptionist and insisting they do a reprint.

12] @abitina: Locuming in a place where they suck at making tea.

13] @danascu: Being caught singing along to the telephone hold music.

14] @DonnaMcCormack1: Being here until I'm 70!

15] @MrDispenser: Answering the phone in the afternoon by saying 'Good morning.'

16] @studentpharmacy: Measuring patients for compression stockings who have smelly feet!

17] @MrDispenser: Being asked to fit a Truss.

18] @MrDispenser: The shutter being half down and me forgetting. Ouch!

19] @MrDispenser: A big prescription one minute to closing time.

20] @Aron2092: Forgetting your lab coat and safety spectacles for a lab practical or professional practice practical.

21] @eilistobin: This lecture will never end. I am hungry.

22] @MrDispenser: Hard to pronounce patient name and there being no one else available for me to palm it off to.

23] @aptaim: Working as a locum in a store without 3G connectivity.

24] @MrDispenser: Not getting any biscuits or chocolates from patients at Christmas.

25] @MrDispenser: Running out of paracetamol.

Giving Feedback

What's the best way of telling someone that they have made you a poor cup of tea?

1] Pharmakeus Prime: Ask them for coffee next time.

2] Abby F: You don't have to tell them. Just looking at the tea in a hurt and horrified way works for me.

3] David F: Ask them if they don't like you.

4] Rachel N: Run to the sink with it at arm's length averting your face which is carrying a look of pure disgust.

5] @checkedshoes: I learnt as a locum pretty much to drink tea as it comes. I avoid coffee in shops I do not know in case it is too strong.

6] Taj: You have to be blunt! I had a girl serve me cold brown milk when I asked for a coffee. I poured it down the sink in front of her.

7] @Pillmanuk: Spraying it out full forced followed by a retching action usually does the job.

8] Darshana T: Spilling it down the sink and making a fresh one.

9] Jo M: Offer to give them a lesson? Say to them "You're a coffee drinker, I take it?"

10] Cam: Shit tea is a sure fire way of getting on any pharmacist's shit list.

11] Natalie D: Tell that person straight. Bad tea is a no no!

12] Shazin M: Don't drink it and go buy one.

13] Michelle D: Take a sip, say ugg and stick out your tongue.

14] Amanda I: Spill it and say oops...then make another...just remember if you take sugar avoid keyboards because the keys stop working and then your waiting times will increase.

15] Si B: Just say *"It's nice, but it's not how my mum makes it."*

16] @cocksparra: *"I asked for a cup of tea, fool, you have brought me pond water."*

17] Aisha A: *"Wow! Did u boil a bar of soap with water in kettle?"*

18] Dinusha H: *"Oh I'm sorry did I ask for a tea? I meant coffee!?"*

19] Rachel S: Drop the cup holding onto your throat gasping *'water...I...need...water'* before grabbing on to the sides of the dispensary and slowly slipping to the floor.

20] Tina A S: I'm in the 'let it go cold or quickly nip out and make yourself another' group.

21] @dressage_diva: You MUST have good tea and good biscuits.

22] Rachel N: I recognise all the tea reactions. I am a bad tea maker!

23] Cathy C: I solve bad tea by making it for everyone when I'm in, then I get it how I like it!

24] Abs: Just pretend to be busy and let the tea go cold. Or say *'you're a coffee person aren't you?'*

25] Nirvair G: This should not happen if you make tea making an essential part of the interview process.

Pens

@josh6h: What are the chances that one day pharmacists will just be paid in pens?

@MrDispenser: Picking up a pen from the pen pot, realising it does not work and putting it back in the pen pot should be a sackable offence.

@MrDispenser: Went to a pharmacy meeting last night and came back with several pens. Yes, pens! I fear a pharmacy stampede now. I'm in witness protection now.

@Xrayser: Patient at reception: *"Can I have a pen?"* Assistant *"Yes - do you need help completing back of script?"* Patient: *"What script?"* (Walks out with pen)

@MrDispenser: Upsetting moment when you give someone a free pen and their only reply is *'What colour is it?'*

@MrDispenser: Our shrinkage is always high due to pen theft.

@frullah_says: I once sellotaped a store alarm/tag onto my pen and it still went missing!

@MrDispenser: That awkward moment when someone at work has stolen your pen and EVERYONE is a suspect.

Stressed: The main small thing I notice that customers do is steal my pen just after I've found a great smooth flowing one, there is nothing worse!

Stressed: I once made the mistake of taking an engraved pen (a gift for graduation) to work on one of my first shifts post-qualifying. It lasted half the day before someone nicked it. I'm still amazed at my own stupidity.

Mr T: I've been to a shop before that keeps the supply of new pens in the CD cabinet.

@frandavi99: I went to work without a pen yesterday and came home with a clicky top!

@MrDispenser: If you ask for my pen so you can sign the back of your prescription, then be prepared for me to watch you like a hawk without blinking.

Joanna B: I don't lend out my pens. I never get them back!

Si B: Get a pen on one of those retractable wires so it pings back when you walk off.

Sal B: I have my name on my pen so I can track it within the pharmacy!

@MrDispenser: Community spirit is alive! Patient has responded to our 'National Pharmacy Pen Shortage' campaign by bringing us a load of bookies pens!

@MrDispenser: Better to have loved and lost than never received that free pen in the first place.

@MrDispenser: I start to write something at work. I walk away. I come back and continue writing and I somehow am writing in a different colour!

Sarah L: I start to write something, I pause for a second, and then go to continue, I have not moved more than 6 inches, and yet there is no pen anywhere to be seen.

Al J: The phantom pen swap - an impressive dispenser's trick, that one.

Terry N: We got to the stage when all the dispensers labelled their pens and I had a special pen that no one dare touch. With the pen situation resolved, we started a continuous game of hide and seek with the scissors and staplers. For all those who work for a certain multiple- these were the days before a 4 letter acronym instructed that such items were attached to the wall with Velcro!

Kim M: Nobody touches my pen unless they want to be searched!

Martin M: Losing a pen only to get home and discover that you put it in some random pocket you never use. I'm the world's least sophisticated unintentional biro smuggler.

Angela C: We used to security-tag our pens that the patients used as we were sick and tired of them being nicked!

Lorraine M: My dispenser and I both chew pens. It's not great when they get swapped.

Sal B: The pen at the counter has been attached to the clipboard with an elastic band. The only time it is changed is when the ink runs out. But customers still try to nab the pen I have in my hand! As for the dispensers my pen is different from the rest...a black Bic biro medium ballpoint...and it sits on my ear under my headscarf, goes everywhere with me! I've had the same pen for a month...record breaker!

Tips for New Doctors

1] Darshana T: Write directions that actually make sense! And no, suppositories cannot be written as "Take two TDS!"

2] Paula B: Hospital Drs, please write the patient's address, it does say name and address and include a quantity to dispense.

3] @MrDispenser: BNF comes out twice a year. There is no reason to keep using one from 2005.

4] @danthedealer: If you issue a prescription with "as directed" on it, please give the patient an idea what that direction is.

5] @danascu: If I can remember how a CD prescription needs to be written, perhaps you can too.

6] @clareylang: Check what strengths/forms CD medicines come in before prescribing.

7] @MrDispenser: Every once in a while, read the prescription before signing.

8] @pillmanuk: Just because the Hospital consultant said prescribe that red traffic lighted drug, you don't have to obey.

9] @MrDispenser: Sign in the box.

10] @lifeonthepharm: Invest in a diary which shows Bank Holidays for writing those tricky instalment scripts.

11] @clareylang: Make sure it is available in the country you're in before you prescribe it.

12] @MrDispenser: There is a magical book called the BNF. Open it and use it.

Motivational Pharmacy Quotes

This was a hashtag started by **@pillmanuk**

1] @PharmakeusEsq: Keep your friends close, but your enemies' closer - by opening up a 100 hour pharmacy next door to them.

2] @GrahamJudas: The only way to do great work is to love what you do. If you haven't found it yet, locum for a bit.

3] @GrahamJudas: Don't be afraid to stand for what you believe in. Even if it means asking for something to be relabelled three times.

4] @MrDispenser: Forget all the reasons it won't work and believe the one reason that it will because the doctor has signed it so must be right.

5] @PharmakeusEsq: Don't sweat the small stuff - we've got some out of date Anhydrol Forte you can have.

6] @MrDispenser: When you say it's hard, you actually mean you can't find the calculator and work out 112-56 in your head.

7] @pillmanuk: The will to win, desire to succeed, urge to reach your full potential. These are the keys that will get you 400 MURs.

8] @MrDispenser: Life is like a CD running balance. You need some negatives in order to appreciate the positives.

9] @pgimmo: The only limit is your own imagination. That and the MUR cap.

10] @MrDispenser: Rule #1 of life. Do what makes YOUR area manager happy.

11] @MrDispenser: Just remember there is someone out there that is more than happy with doing less MURs than you.

12] @pillmanuk: If you're going through hell, you're in pharmacy.

13] @PharmakeusEsq: Success is the ability to go from one deprived run-down pharmacy to another with no loss of enthusiasm.

14] @MrDispenser: I am thankful for all of those who said NO to me. It's because of them I'm locuming 70 miles from where I live.

15] @jasonpeett: When they say 100 hours they actually don't mean Earth Hours. That would be silly.

16] @MrDispenser: I don't regret the things I've done, I regret the things I didn't do when I was still signed in as the RP.

17] @pillmanuk: If at first you don't succeed, bang in a 100 hour contract.

Two Worst Words in Pharmacy

1] **@edantjam:** No tea!

2] **@satspatel:** New FY1s.

3] **@hollymack:** Handwriting labels.

4] **@kelbel69696969:** Spines down.

5] **@DressageDivaDee:** Short staffed.

6] **@PharmakeusEsq:** New Dosette.

7] **@DressageDivaDee:** On quota.

8] **Catherine** D: Missing keys.

9] **@rosey_aa:** Customer complaint.

10] **@alilvshk:** Missing prescription.

11] **@MrDispenser:** Handwritten prescription.

12] **@ericalee87:** Gluten free.

13] **@boo2112:** Specific brand.

14] **@desmondie:** Specials invoice.

15] **@hippymoo:** Patient return.

16] **@katos1981:** Date check.

17] **@ode79:** Fridge alarm.

18] @LouiseBrueton: Shipping order.

19] @medicineman61: Drivers late.

20] @MrDispenser: Taxi waiting.

21] Tracey C: Empty box.

22] @CrazyRxMan: Ready yet?

23] @lcd967: Controlled drugs.

24] @medicineman61: Double booked.

25] @KezMartin_x: Special order.

26] @camshim: Call helpdesk.

27] @jobiwhan: Awkward customer.

28] Cleverestcookie : Spilt Winchester.

29] @jobiwhan: Hungover locum.

30] @medicineman61: Please reorder.

31] @cerirhian: On call.

32] @MrDispenser: Calculator broken.

33] @MrDispenser: Newly qualified.

34] @PatelSuk: Branded generic.

35] @Cleverestcookie: Extemporaneous preparation.

36] @BottSlot: Emergency Supply.

Don't date a pharmacist

1] @MrDispenser: Every time they see any kind of reps, they shake them vigorously in case any pens fall loose.

2] @_Amberetto: They'll ruin every medical drama by shouting about the lack of pharmacists.

3] @HelenPoots: Larder alphabetised (apart from generic beans under "h" for Heinz).

4] @TwandyLaw: Post-it notes. Pharmaceutical branded post-it notes everywhere.

5] @MrDispenser: Every time they pour you a drink, they watch you drink it all and record it in a book.

6] @Bridgetradomski: They get grumpy if you ask for banana flavour milkshake because you won't drink any other flavour.

7] @angelalexander: Why not? They are patient lovers.

8] @Cleverestcookie: You may fall in love, and then... WWHAM!

9] @EmilyJaneBond82: They are notoriously poor sleepers, whimpering 'manufacturer cannot supply' and lashing out.

10] @EmilyJaneBond82: Your drinks cupboard will be scrupulously date checked and filled with pointless scratch cards.

11] @MrDispenser: They only half listen to your conversation. They are also listening to the reality TV show to join in the conversation at work.

12] @mrs_p_face: They give you inferior gifts for birthdays and Christmas and insist they are just as good as the expensive ones.

13] @iain_rough: When you go to meet them for lunch you'll find a sign informing you to come back in an hour.

14] @MrDispenser: They will offer you a hot drink but then get their tech to make it.

15] @MrDispenser: They will steal your pens.

The End

If you have enjoyed this book then please let me know via mrdispenser@hotmail.co.uk, tweet me @MrDispenser or post on my Facebook page. Please also send me your funny pharmacy stories and tell your pharmacy friends too.

Sometimes, it's the little things that brighten up the day.....

@ashyhanvidge: Loving work today. Locum pharmacist let us turn the radio up full blast and dance around the dispensary.

Printed in Great Britain
by Amazon